Psychotherapist and hypnotherapist Susan Hepburn is a leading weight-loss expert with clinics in London's Harley Street, New York, LA and Europe. She has over 23 years' experience and her clients range from A-list actors to rock stars and sports personalities. She accompanied the England football squad to the Japan World Cup and has made many TV appearances. She is also the author of *F*** Diets* and the Amazon bestseller *Stop Smoking in One Hour*.

Praise for Susan Hepburn

Hypnodieting with Susan Hepburn is 'the hottest new diet craze to emerge from the States'.

Marie Claire

Susan Hepburn's Hypnodiet is 'the hottest body trend of 2009'.

Grazia

'The secret to Lily Allen's dramatic weight loss has been revealed – hypnotherapy . . . with Susan Hepburn.'

Daily Mail

'Lily Allen slimmed down with the help of Susan Hepburn, an accredited hypnotherapist and psychotherapist.'

US Weekly

Hypno DIET

LOSE WEIGHT, FEEL FABULOUS –
THE STRESS-FREE WAY

SUSAN HEPBURN

piatkus

I would like to thank the many people who have helped me
in so many ways with this book.

PIATKUS

First published in Great Britain in 2010 by Piatkus
Reprinted 2010

A CIP catalogue record for this book
is available from the British Library

ISBN 978-0-7499-5235-8

Typeset in Sabon by M Rules
Printed and bound in Great Britain by
Clays Ltd, St Ives plc

Papers used by Piatkus are natural, renewable and
recyclable products sourced from well-managed forests and certified
in accordance with the rules of the Forest Stewardship Council.

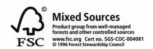

Mixed Sources
Product group from well-managed
forests and other controlled sources
www.fsc.org   Cert no. SGS-COC-004081
© 1996 Forest Stewardship Council
FSC

Piatkus
An imprint of
Little, Brown Book Group
100 Victoria Embankment
London EC4Y 0DY

An Hachette UK Company
www.hachette.co.uk

www.piatkus.co.uk

Contents

Introduction

This is not a diet. Diets just don't work. It's not a miracle cure either – although I hope you'll see miraculous results. It's not a fad; I won't be giving you tricks or gimmicks, or asking you to exist on cabbage soup or crispbreads. In fact, there won't be any deprivation, guilt or pain at all. Hypnodiet is simple: it allows you to make peace with food and with your body – for ever.

This book and accompanying CD will teach you new habits that will last a lifetime. You'll learn to eat when you're hungry and stop when you're full. This isn't traumatic or difficult, and it doesn't take loads of willpower. With Hypnodiet, when you're not hungry you simply will not want to eat. You'll learn to make healthy choices and to take regular exercise, to embrace exercise and view it as an essential part of your daily life, rather than an optional extra. Best of all, you'll start to feel good about yourself and about your body. It doesn't matter how much or how little you have to lose, it is simply what matters to you that is important, and in most cases it is more about being able to take control of your eating habits. And what's more, you don't need a personal trainer or private chef to see results.

Over the past 23 years as a weight-loss expert I've seen thousands of people at my clinics in New York, LA, Europe and London's Harley Street. I work with anyone: from celebrity A-listers and the England football squad to countless people with ordinary lives – men and women of all ages and backgrounds.

I first saw Paula, 24, who works in the City, in October 2007. She was a size 18. She wanted to be a size 10, but she was convinced that she'd never lose weight. She said she'd read about me and that it had given her hope. She told me that people would say to her, 'It's such a shame [about your weight] – you've got a really pretty face', and her father would say, 'You'll be stunning when you lose weight.' Sometimes he'd comment, 'You're so fat, you should be ashamed of yourself. You'll never get anyone to marry you. Why are you doing this to yourself?' Her self-esteem was at rock bottom.

By February 2008, when she came back for her third – and final – Hypnodiet session, she had dropped to a size 14. 'Everyone I work with has commented that they can't believe how it's changed my personality, how much confidence I have now,' she told me, with a huge smile. She had changed her job, within the same company, to one with more face-to-face client contact, and she has had her first ever boyfriend. 'Whereas before I didn't like to be seen,' she said, 'now I just want to be around people. And I can't stop smiling. I'm really chatty, whereas before I would just want to hide.'

Paula confessed that she still had the odd fear. 'Sometimes I think, *Ooh, what if it doesn't work; what if I put all the weight back on again*, but then I start thinking, *No, it's going to work.*'

I recently saw Paula for an unrelated issue. She looks fabulous. She's a size 10 and almost unrecognisable, not just because of her weight loss but also because of her enormous confidence and energy. She is brimming with happiness.

What all my clients have in common when they first come to me, whether they are famous or not, is a sense of despair. Deep down they fear they'll never be the weight and size they want to be.

They have often tried virtually every diet available, and even own a small library of diet books, forever seeking that seemingly elusive solution to their weight problem. They've probably tried everything from extremely low-calorie diets to scary detox plans – often losing and gaining tens of pounds/ kilos in the process. They end up bigger than they were to begin with. Often they punish themselves for this – what they see as 'failure'. They feel helpless and believe that they lack willpower. One guy said, 'When I wake up, I think about food; when I go to bed, I think about food.' He certainly isn't alone. Food becomes an obsession – a very unhappy one.

Even when they're 'thin' they can't enjoy the lost inches because they're so paranoid and anxious that they might pile the weight back on again. Not surprisingly, their relationship with food is fraught.

If I've learned one thing over the years, it's that dieting is futile. I'll talk about this in more detail in Chapter 1. But it's important to know that your diet trials can – and will – stop, right now. By buying this book you've taken the first step to enjoying food and your body in a balanced, healthy way for the rest of your life. Throughout this book I'll be giving you information and tips on how to establish a healthy lifestyle that suits you, and is sustainable.

SO, HOW DOES IT WORK?

For many people the word 'hypnotism' brings to mind gimmicky TV shows where a charismatic Svengali-type figure 'controls' people, getting them to do funny, and often embarrassing, things. This couldn't be further from what I do. Hypnosis is actually a very subtle technique. I don't 'put people under' or play tricks with the mind.

I'm simply going to teach you techniques that allow you to reach a state of deep, but lucid, relaxation. Ultimately, you are in charge of this process, not me. When you are in this state of deep relaxation (hypnosis), it is possible to bypass the conscious mind and reach the more 'suggestible' subconscious. This part of your mind holds the deep-rooted habits, beliefs and impulses that undermine your best intentions.

With Hypnodiet you'll 'reprogramme' your subconscious mind. This isn't a wild and unrealistic claim. Hypnosis can be a powerful tool for behavioural change. And the human mind is capable of unbelievable things. This is why, as a psychologist, I began to use hypnosis techniques in the first place. There are well-documented cases of people using self-hypnosis to undergo surgery or dental treatment without anaesthetic. Hypnosis can be used for drug-free childbirth ('hypnobirthing'). One clinical trial even found self-hypnosis could reduce the symptoms of hay fever. The techniques aren't magic – they just allow people to distance themselves from pain and to remove associated feelings of anxiety and fear. It works in a similar way with food.

I liken it to deleting unwanted files from a computer. First you remove from your subconscious mind the emotional associations that cause you to eat when you are not hungry (behaviours such as comfort eating or eating because of boredom, stress or tiredness). Next, you reprogramme your mind with healthy and positive attitudes to food and exercise.

To do this, I'll be asking you to follow a straightforward programme of short, daily meditations. I'll guide you through these on the CD that comes with this book. Don't worry: this won't involve any special skills or chanting. By meditations, I just mean quiet sessions in which you'll learn to relax your body and mind.

For this to work you're going to need to set aside about

20 minutes of each day. That's not much of a commitment when you think about it. During these meditations you'll identify your problematic eating habits. You'll then replace them with patterns of behaviour that allow you to lose weight, without feeling you are being deprived of anything at all. Through the power of suggestion I will guide you and do most of this work for you.

The other concept central to Hypnodiet is 'mindfulness'. Mindfulness is a highly effective psychological tool, gaining ground both in popular culture and mainstream psychology (clinical trials show that mindfulness-based stress-reduction programmes can help with anything from pain management in cancer patients to long-term depression). Hypnodiet is not a mindfulness course, but it will certainly encourage you to eat 'mindfully': to really savour food, so that you enjoy and get the most out of eating, becoming more aware of what you put into your body, and therefore making healthier choices.

Most people I see have lost touch with their bodies, they just don't know what it is to eat 'normally' any more. 'I eat massive portions,' one client recently told me, 'but I never know when I'm full.' With Hypnodiet, you'll learn to eat what you want, but in moderation, because you will – at long last – feel satisfied. My method promotes a mindful awareness that will permanently change your attitude towards food.

I also encourage you to keep a food diary. This will help you to unpick the emotional associations you have with food and to understand your 'triggers' – the feelings that make you eat when you're not hungry. (Studies show that keeping a daily food diary can help weight loss.)

Finally, I recommend that you put away your bathroom scales – and ideally ditch them entirely. Weighing yourself can become a stressful obsession. Do you really need to know your weight every day? Why bother? You'll know it's working by how your clothes fit and feel, and how your body feels. Throwing out the scales will seriously boost your 'feel-good factor' and this, in turn, will help to motivate you.

Hypnodiet is not just for today, or next week, or until you can fit into your skinny jeans – it's for ever. This is not a life sentence, it's liberating! You'll never have to fear going out to dinner any more, or beat yourself up for wanting some chocolate or a piece of cheese. My philosophy is 'everything in moderation'. The 'moderation' part may have been too hard to stick to before, but it isn't now. Moderation and healthy eating – not deprivation and feast/famine behaviour – are the cornerstones of Hypnodiet. Any good nutritionist will tell you that this is the way to eat for life.

Hypnodiet will enable you to lose weight and keep it off. I've seen thousands of people succeed – people who are vastly overweight, people who have been stuck in dreadful eating patterns for years, who have tried everything and have come to me as a last resort.

As you do your daily meditations, you will replace the

self-criticism with self-acceptance. Your self-esteem will soar as you begin to see what you can achieve, and how painless it is. Very soon, you'll find that you enjoy your food, and eat to satisfy your hunger. You will begin to view food as an enjoyable fuel for your body.

Hypnodiet isn't rocket science. It's no secret how to lose those inches. It's the simplicity of my method that makes it so effective and appealing. You have all the skills you need right here, right now: in your mind. So, find a quiet spot, open your mind and start the journey that will lead you to the shape you want to be.

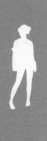

Around 96 per cent of my clients lose weight and keep it off. Hypnodiet teaches you to have a normal, healthy relationship with food – without guilt.

Chapter 1

ARE YOU BORED WITH BEING ON A DIET?

You've probably gathered by now that I'm not a big diet fan. You may be disappointed to hear this, having bought a book called *Hypnodiet*. But, despite its name, my method is designed to liberate you from diet hell, not just now but always. The name Hypnodiet, in fact, springs from the understanding that to get your attention I have to dangle that carrot. And you *will* lose weight – permanently – if you work with me. But in reality Hypnodiet is not a regime at all. I won't be telling you about forbidden foods or calorie counting, I won't be exhorting you to have willpower, and you're not going to be weighing and measuring yourself.

Here's why.

LEARNING TO FORGET THE 'D' WORD

Through 23 years of research, studying eating habits and listening to people's stories – their disastrous attempts at dieting, their food battles and their emotional ordeals – I know that the key to staying at a healthy weight is to put all thoughts of 'dieting' out of your mind.

Diets only *appear* to work. Some work better than others, but they aren't sustainable and they rarely tackle the root cause of the problem: the mind.

I've heard some horror stories over the years. And these stories are getting worse as more diets flood the market. The bottom line is that we now live in a 'supersize' culture. Food – most of it fast and unhealthy – is available on every corner, every hour of the day or night. We also get far less exercise than previous generations. Experts call this the 'obesity epidemic', and it's getting worse all the time.

THE PAIN OF DESPERATION

Over the years I've seen a change. Despite the diet choices out there, people who come to me are *more* desperate, not less. They'll try to lose weight at virtually any cost. I regularly see people who have been on diets that are so restrictive they pose a serious health hazard. I've treated people who have spent their life savings on gastric bands, stomach stapling and liposuction – sometimes with life-threatening consequences.

★ **Case Study:** Caroline

ONE OF MY CLIENTS, 47-YEAR-OLD CAROLINE, had a gastric band fitted just before Christmas one year. She thought she could recuperate over the holidays. On her first night at home she experienced excruciating stomach pains and was rushed to hospital where she underwent emergency surgery to have the band removed. She spent that Christmas in intensive care while her family, including her sister who had come all the way from Australia, sat helplessly by, waiting to hear whether she would survive. Caroline now has an ugly scar across her abdomen, is thousands of pounds poorer, and her doctor said she's lucky to be alive. All she wanted was an end to her weight battles.

I am not suggesting that everyone who has a gastric band fitted will experience Caroline's disastrous results; however, this possible danger cannot be overlooked.

With Hypnodiet, Caroline finally found what she wanted. She is losing weight steadily and healthily, and feels great.

THE PROOF OF THOUSANDS

You too can achieve your target size and maintain it without any desperate measures. You probably don't believe this, but it's true. I've helped thousands of people to do just this.

Virtually everyone I see is cynical to begin with. They've

tried virtually every diet going; they start off enthusiastic, full of hope that the chosen diet will be 'the one', but they all end up the same: in dismal failure.

★ **Case Study:** Allie

ALLIE, A MARKETING EXECUTIVE, is a classic example of a failed dieter who came to me in despair.

'I followed one diet that seemed to be successful and lost 3 stone, then I put it back on quicker than I had lost it. It was quite alarming actually; it was as though someone was pumping me up. I had everything when I was on the diet: hair loss, my periods stopped, I thought I was going into early menopause and I am only 35 – I still want to have children. But I didn't care because I wanted to lose the weight so badly. Now I have put it all back on again and more besides. I hated myself and blamed myself all the time.'

A COMPLETELY DIFFERENT APPROACH

People like Allie come to me because they've got a hunch that what I'm offering could be different – and they've got to try *something*. But at the same time they're asking themselves, 'Why should this work? Why am I bothering?'

Then they see the weight beginning to drop off. The effect of this is often profound. Many of my clients – men and women of all ages – become very emotional, there are tears of relief when they realise that this is actually working. For the first time they feel different about themselves. Recently, a woman wrote to thank me: 'Since your treatment I've had smaller portions, eaten very healthily and have been exercising – all unheard of for me, totally unheard of,' she said. 'I worry sometimes that it will stop working, but then it feels different and I know I can do this!'

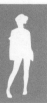

Achieve your target size and stay there – without going on a diet ever again.

Virtually everyone tells me that they don't want to follow diets any more; they are tired of them and upset to have gone through so much for nothing, as they are back to square one: still battling those inches.

WHY DIETS DON'T WORK

There is a vast amount of scientific research that demonstrates just how pointless – even harmful – radical dieting can be. For a start, diets are generally only effective when you are on them, being monitored, or monitoring yourself, all the time. This just isn't sustainable for most of us in the real world. Equally, a daily eating regime that leaves you hungry, irritable, and even feeling ill, is never going to be a way to eat for life.

Deprivation is no way to live. And it is certainly not good for your body or your mind.

HOW IT ALL GOES WRONG

This is where 'yo-yo' dieting behaviour kicks in. You'll know the drill by now: you start counting points, measuring foods, drinking only fluids or eating dull – or perhaps unpalatable – foods. Generally, you feel hungry most of the time. You may manage to lose some weight because you have cut calories. For a few months, sometimes more, you may look marvellous – everyone compliments you. But then the weight starts to creep back on.

You can't resist the foods you've been deprived of for so long – usually the ones you love the most, which are often the 'bad fat' variety. Some days you gorge, other days you starve yourself. You begin to feel guilty or panicky about your 'sins' and you start mentally beating yourself up.

Then you begin to eat more, out of rebellion, sadness, self-hatred or the desire for comfort – there can be any number of emotional reasons why people eat (I'll be unpicking this in Chapter 2). Before you know it, the weight is all back again.

You then eat even more because you're so unhappy about

this weight gain. Then you're even heavier than you were to begin with. You can't fit into your 'fat clothes'. Finally, in desperation, you go on another – sometimes even more radical – diet.

The result is that you go through life one step away from a diet at any time.

★ **Case Study:** Eloise

ONE OF MY CLIENTS, ELOISE, 34, used to be a swimmer. One thoughtless comment from a trainer when she was 15 years old threw her into a lifetime of dieting. 'I am definitely a serial dieter,' she said, 'always on diets'. But over the years, despite all her attempts to lose weight, the pounds have piled on. Now, she hardly recognises herself. *'Recently, old friends wanted to meet up and I thought,* Oh crikey! Three stone later, I can't meet them. They haven't seen me since I put all this weight on.'

Over the years this yo-yo behaviour adds up to an awful lot of heartache, not to mention pounds gained and lost (which is, incidentally, harmful for the body, putting a strain on the heart and disrupting the metabolism so that it becomes harder to lose weight than ever before).

In other words, the diet industry is a complete and utter con. This is why my method will banish diets from your life, for good.

Beware: most diets will fail you

Scientific research demonstrates that diets rarely live up to their inflated claims. They tell you they have the magical formula: all you have to do is avoid eating carbs, or eat according to your blood type, or eat like prehistoric man, or eat only at certain times of the day, or combine only certain foods – and then the weight will miraculously drop off.

It's all nonsense. The only way to lose weight is to consume fewer calories than you burn off ('calories in' versus 'calories out'). You may do this for a short while on these diets – they all rely on getting you to eat fewer calories, whatever they say – but at what cost?

When scientists at Stanford University in the US recently compared four popular diets they were flabbergasted to see how little weight participants actually lost. Those on the low-carb diet, for instance, on average lost only just over 4.5kg (10lb), from a starting weight averaging 86kg (13½st/190lb). Those on the other three diets, on average, lost less than 2.7kg (6lb). This is not a huge loss to show for hours of agonising and self-denial. I'm sure you've had similar experiences yourself.

But here's the truth: countless reputable scientific studies have found that only a small minority of dieters manage to achieve sustained weight loss. The majority regain all the weight, plus a little extra for good measure.

IT CAN BE SO HARD TO DO WHAT YOU KNOW YOU SHOULD

You probably know all too well the 'theory' of how to lose weight. It's no secret. You know what to eat and do, but you just can't stick to it. Some of the people I see even have a personal chef, either at home or in the office, but they still can't eat healthily, like Eleanor for example.

★ **Case Study:** Eleanor

ELEANOR, 52, told me:

'The chef cooks for my family, preparing fruit plates and really healthy meals. I even order the food for my family – all organic, lots of fish and vegetables. I want them to have a balanced healthy diet, but I never eat any of it. I just eat crap. I also drink three large bottles of diet cola a day!'

When Eleanor came back to me for her follow-up session she expressed absolute amazement that she hadn't had, or wanted, any diet cola at all since our first meeting. She was eating healthy meals with her family and loving it. She told me:

'I feel liberated!'

YOUR TOOLS FOR SUCCESS

I'm going to give you the tools to liberate yourself. It won't be a matter of 'sticking' to anything, because eating healthily and in moderation will become second nature to you – a way of life. You'll want to do it. You won't have to deprive yourself of anything and you'll remove the guilt and pain associated with eating. You'll do this by reprogramming your mind.

This isn't a crazy claim. I actually see most clients for only two or three sessions, although they have to practise the meditations on their own. Hypnosis is fast and effective. You'll immediately see your behaviour change from 'I need a snack' to 'I'd like a snack, but I don't need one, so I'll wait', or 'I don't want a snack at all'. The impulse to have unhealthy snacks may be there occasionally, but the connection between impulse and action is not made. This will give you a sense of calm and confidence. That's something diets never do. It will also banish anxiety and self-doubt – most people say that they actually enjoy the Hypnodiet process.

> *You will start to see results from the moment you listen to the CD.*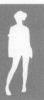

★ **Case Study:** Jenna

'I have been absolutely brilliant with the self-hypnosis,' Jenna told me in her follow-up appointment the other day.

'I have done it twice a day. I absolutely do it every day and I

feel like it is working – it's quite amazing. It's such a change for me to follow a programme and stick to it.'

Hypnodiet is not a quick fix, though. You do have to make an effort – but it's a pleasant, life-enhancing effort to make.

THE KEY IS IN THE CD

It's very important to listen to the CD daily until you reach your desired size, then continue listening just twice a week in order to maintain your fabulous new body. It is possible for *anyone* to find 20 minutes each day, and what could be more important than your future health and happiness? By listening to the CD each day, and following my instructions, you will create new and permanent patterns in your subconscious that will change your relationship with your body for ever.

What you can expect

- From the outset, after listening to the CD, you will find that you want to eat healthier foods.
- You will stop eating when you've reached that 'had enough to eat' feeling.
- You will reduce – or even eliminate – the impulse to snack.
- You will see what a positive part of your daily life exercise can be.

---

*Hypno*DIET tip
How to establish a routine

Set aside 20 minutes at the same time each day – perhaps just after waking or during the day – for your meditation with the CD. Make this part of your routine: same time each day, every day. We all have busy lives and huge 'to-do' lists, but don't let this be at the bottom of yours. If you say to yourself, 'I'll do it later' you probably won't, but if you set aside a regular slot, it will become easier and easier. Before you know it you'll be hooked on this valuable 'me time'. Putting the CD on your iPod or MP3 player allows you to continue this, even while on business travel or vacations.

You may decide to read the book first and then listen to the CD. However, you may be so excited to get started that you decide to listen to the CD first and then read the remainder of the book afterwards. You can do whichever way suits you best. However, please do not skip the book altogether, as this is an equally important part of the programme.

It's that simple. No gimmicks. No fads. Say goodbye to diets permanently.

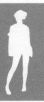

Remember that it's important to listen to the CD every day until you have reached your target size. You may then find that listening to the CD just twice a week will be all that you need to maintain your desired size.

Chapter 2

HOW DID I GET THIS WAY?

Many of my clients have developed such a complex and destructive relationship with food that they have lost touch, entirely, with what it means to eat 'normally'. People's ideas about food can become distorted. Many people use it as a reward – a comfort – or they deny themselves food as a punishment.

What is more, we live in a very commercial world. Magazines, movies, television and other media constantly tell us that we must be thin at all costs. Being thin, they suggest, is the key to happiness. Anything other than that and you won't fit in; you can never be beautiful. Instead, you belong with the other world: the 'fat world'. This is somehow a lesser place, less successful, less beautiful, less glamorous and less desirable.

It is easy to become obsessed, and to feel worthless.

THE DEVASTATION OF AN EATING DISORDER

Eating disorders work in a similar way. If you are a young girl with a large circle of friends, some of whom are either anorexic or bulimic, or both, then by developing an eating disorder you, too, can 'fit in'. Take Gemma, for example.

★ **Case Study:** *Gemma*

I ALWAYS REMEMBER GEMMA, A 32-YEAR-OLD who had been suffering from anorexia and bulimia since she was 13. She had returned to boarding school after the summer break and a friend asked about her rounded tummy. Gemma said she had been eating lots of ice cream and chocolate and couldn't get rid of it. 'Oh it's easy,' said her friend, 'just make yourself sick after every meal and then you can eat whatever you want without getting fat.' *What an easy solution*, Gemma thought . . .

A staggering 19 years later, Gemma was still battling with the demons that had begun that day. When she saw me, she was totally obsessed with food and being slim – still pursuing that firm, flat stomach, which seemed to evade her. To make it worse, she had chosen a boyfriend who disapproved of her gaining any weight. He made it quite clear that he was not attracted to her if she did. She lived in constant fear that he might leave her one day.

After doing Hypnodiet, Gemma's world has completely

changed. She no longer makes herself sick, she has a balanced, normal relationship with food. She has also gained in confidence – she can even enjoy the occasional chocolate bar these days.

In our sessions we addressed Gemma's body image, her self-esteem and self-worth. She learned how to love herself unconditionally, whether her body seemed perfect or flawed to her. To Gemma's delight, and to mine too, she found a new boyfriend, who loves her for who she is, and they are soon to be married.

For those with eating disorders, it can seem impossible to imagine life without thinking 24/7 about food. But it is possible. Gemma thought she'd never be free of her obsessions – and she is. You can be free too.

> *You can love yourself unconditionally – free of negative associations with food.*

A PATTERN FROM CHILDHOOD

It is quite common for these patterns of thought and behaviour to go right back to childhood, as we can see in the case of Leyla.

★ **Case Study:** Leyla

LEYLA, IN HER FORTIES, works part-time as a paediatrician, and the rest of the time she cares for her 12-year-old twin daughters. 'I have been binge eating since I was a kid,' she told me at our first session.

'I will buy a packet of muffins and eat them all in one go. Or I'll buy packets of croissants or scones . . . anything that can be bought in bulk and looks normal in my shopping bag, so no one will suspect me. I then hate myself even more and feel so guilty – and thank goodness no one has caught me.'

Leyla traces her issues around food all the way back to childhood – to the messages she got from those she loved.

'At 12 years of age I loathed myself. I was fat, fat, fat. I was always told that I was fat. My father said I was fat, my mother said I was fat.'

When she came to see me she told me how difficult her life had become:

'My kids drive me nuts. They have always been challenging – there is chaos and mess all the time. I often feel so angry and resentful – I think this has a lot to do with my relationship with food. If I get annoyed with my husband, I just shovel food down like there's no tomorrow. I have made myself sick a few times in my life, I hate doing it but I hate my body and my eating even more.'

The kind of childhood 'conditioning' Leyla experienced can have a profound and lasting psychological impact on your eating habits. Add the stresses and strains of adult life, and it is all too easy to turn to food for comfort or escape.

FOOD: ESCAPE FROM THE PAIN

Anger, stress, anxiety, pain – all these emotions, and more, can cause you to turn to food for solace. Like so many people, Leyla's stressful life contributed directly to her compulsive overeating. She told me that she felt pulled in all directions.

'ONLY JOKING'

Constant criticism and negativity from others can cause untold emotional damage. Eating disorders and obesity can be triggered by the seemingly 'harmless' behaviour of those around you: a teasing brother, father or school friends, for example. (Brothers just love to tease, and sisters make an easy target – I have seen countless women whose eating problems stem from sibling teasing.)

The self-destructive behaviour that results from such teasing, criticism and negative comments can last a lifetime.

Most parents would be horrified if they realised that their throwaway comments had caused unbelievable and lasting problems in their children. In psychology, this is called 'classical conditioning'. But classical conditioning can equally be therapeutic. You can 'recondition yourself' so that you change your own thought processes, eliminating fears or distorted thoughts. By doing this, you will be able to enjoy a normal healthy relationship with food.

> *You can change your self-destructive behaviour by listening to your inner voice. The Hypnodiet CD will help you to develop this voice, and to strengthen it.*

TRAPPED IN A VICIOUS CYCLE

Like Leyla, you may find that eating is a cycle of guilt and self-loathing; that it can be fear and pleasure and pain all mixed together. You may find that it is virtually impossible to simply eat when you are hungry and stop when you are full. You may have got to the stage where you can't listen to your body any more because its messages have become too mixed and confusing. And so you find yourself reaching for packets of crisps, biscuits and chocolate, or microwave dinners, out of boredom, pain or anxiety. You eat even though your mind is saying you 'shouldn't'.

Or perhaps, more often than not, you really don't know why you're eating – you just are.

LOSING A SENSE OF REALITY

You find that you can't stop, even when you've had enough. Sometimes you don't know whether you've had enough or not – the signals from your brain have become too confused.

You might skip meals – perhaps you never have breakfast, or you skip lunch, feeling guilty because of a blowout the night before – but then you overeat again at 6.00 p.m. because you're starving. On a diet, you measure how well you are doing by how many meals you have managed to skip and not feel hungry.

You might go on fasts and detoxes – but, after them, you will binge destructively. You probably have 'forbidden' or 'sinful' foods. You may cut them out entirely for a while, and then eat them in abundance as a kind of backlash.

This behaviour, for some people, becomes extreme – life-threatening, in fact.

★ **Case Study:** Deborah

DEBORAH, 35, an artist, came to me because her battles with food were seriously jeopardising her health.

'I am diabetic so I know I should eat regular meals. But if I feel fat I'll either go on a detox or I just won't eat. I remember *someone once said that I had a lollipop head, and they meant that my body was so skinny and malnourished that my head seemed out of proportion. I never think about food when I am happy but if I am unhappy I'll think about food all the time, or I make sure that I don't have food at all. It's ridiculous because my mother died of a diabetic coma, but I can't seem to stop myself.'*

FOOD BECOMES THE *ONLY* THING

When your relationship with food has become abnormal in this way, it is easy to become obsessed with eating. Food can dominate your life.

The majority of people I have helped over the past 23 years have described themselves as being obsessed with food. Many have a poor and negative relationship with their bodies and with eating, and they have a distorted body image. This obsession can lead to bingeing, purging, starving and addiction. You may be surprised to hear the word 'addiction' related to food here; after all, each one of us needs to eat every day. But many of us do indeed have an addiction to food, and there are a number of associated serious diseases connected with it. Whereas there are measures in place to help people deal with other common addictions, such as smoking, drug abuse and alcohol, an addiction to food is not so easily recognised or helped.

★ **Case Study:** Derek

DEREK, 39, an actor, said:

'If someone says we're not going to eat until a certain time, I panic. I am constantly thinking about food – what I'll eat next, when, how. It's ruling my life.'

He then followed Hypnodiet because he had put on several kilos and was convinced that his weight was stopping him from getting acting roles.

There are numerous reasons why people develop an unhealthy relationship with food, but when they do, it can impact on their entire lives and the lives of those around them.

★ **Case Study:** Angela

ANGELA, 52, a solicitor, wanted to lose 25kg (4st/56lb). Her negative body image, she said, was seriously threatening her relationship with her husband:

'My marriage is not particularly good at the best of times. My husband gets on my nerves a lot – he is constantly nagging for sex, but I don't feel good about myself and my body, so I don't want to have sex. I don't even want him to see me naked. It's all so awful. I feel that my life is a mess.'

When your eating is unbalanced in this way, and your feelings about your body – your entire being – become so negative, the pleasure of food can then become so clouded that it is hardly a pleasure at all.

ARE YOU OBSESSED WITH FOOD?

Take some time to complete this short questionnaire to discover your relationship with food. Answer the questions openly and honestly – you are the only person who will see the answers.

		Yes	No
1	Do you think about food when you are not hungry?	☐	☐
2	Do you sometimes skip meals, as you think it will help you to lose weight?	☐	☐
3	Are you unhappy with your body shape and size?	☐	☐
4	Are you anxious at the thought of someone seeing you naked?	☐	☐
5	Are you afraid of becoming fat?	☐	☐
6	Do you ever avoid going out because you feel fat and unattractive?	☐	☐
7	Do you weigh yourself more than once a day?	☐	☐
8	Do you feel out of control in that you eat a whole packet of biscuits rather than just one or two?	☐	☐
9	Are you constantly changing from one fad diet to another and become impatient when a diet doesn't seem to be working fast enough?	☐	☐

		Yes	No
10	Do you ever eat in secret?	☐	☐
11	Do you measure your happiness by how slim you are and how little you can eat without feeling nauseous?	☐	☐
12	Do you avoid events when you know food will be there?	☐	☐
13	Do you binge and then feel anxious and bad about yourself?	☐	☐
14	Have you ever tried dieting methods in desperation, which you would feel too embarrassed to tell anyone about, such as laxatives, enemas, vomiting, diet pills, gastric bands, and so on?	☐	☐
15	Do you become anxious and feel guilty sometimes after you have eaten a treat?	☐	☐
16	Are you convinced that you will never be slim and happy?	☐	☐

Score 1 for each 'yes' answer.

Total score: ☐

Over 4: Your relationship with food is becoming unbalanced.
Over 8: You're on your way to becoming obsessed with food.
Over 15: Your emotional well-being is becoming severely affected, but Hypnodiet can change this.

THE POWER OF GUILT

Guilt is a hugely destructive emotion. It can dominate your whole relationship with food. If you are trapped in over-eating, food and guilt will go hand in hand. The pleasure you get from eating is constantly complicated by a voice saying, 'I shouldn't be doing this', 'This is so fattening', 'This is forbidden', 'This is going to undo all my good work . . .' and so on. I have listened to many plaintive cries from brides, who say, 'I know that if I carry on eating in this destructive way, my wedding gown won't fit, yet I cannot stop. I even tell myself this, while I'm stuffing my face, but I still don't stop.'

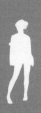

Hypnodiet helps you to deal with your food obsessions and anxiety, allowing you to enjoy a normal healthy relationship with food.

Terrible cycles of behaviour can grow out of guilty thoughts around food. You eat; you feel guilty; then you eat even more, thinking to yourself, *I have no restraint. I've blown it now. I can't stop.* This constant soundtrack is not just tiresome and upsetting it's also destructive – warping your ability to eat what your body needs and being unable to enjoy it.

The good news is that you can cut off your guilt sound-track *right now*.

Hypnodiet will liberate you from guilt once and for all, allowing you to eat the small piece of chocolate, the cupcake, the small chunk of cheese – or whatever you fancy to eat – without feeling that you have sinned or are weak, or that you have 'blown it'.

> *Hypnodiet allows you to break the connection between eating and guilty thoughts.*

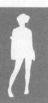

HOW TO WORK OUT YOUR EMOTIONAL TRIGGERS RELATING TO FOOD

Set aside five or ten minutes and sit down with a pen and paper. Try to answer the following two groups of questions as honestly as you can. They will help you to understand more about your emotional relationship with food and help you to understand yourself more.

A: Where did it all begin?

1 Was your body image partly formed by comments someone made to you?

2 Was it a particular event that made you feel bad about yourself?

3   Did the comment make you dislike that person at the time?

4   Did your eating issues begin with a childhood trauma such as a divorce? Emotional abuse? Or bereavement?

5   Did your eating issues begin later in life as a result of a trauma – a relationship break-up, job loss, exam failure, depression or another kind of crisis?

6   Do you feel that you have always been overweight, even as a small child?

7   How old were you when your weight issues began?

8   How old were you when you started your dieting career?

B: Your eating patterns

1   Do you try to skip as many meals as possible?

2   Do you count calories and try to eat as few as possible every day?

3   Do you have days when you binge and days of abstinence?

4   Do you constantly start new diets?

5   Do you know the calorific values of most types of food?

6   Do you have 'forbidden' or 'sinful' foods?

7   Do you feel preoccupied by food – constantly planning when and what you will eat next?

8   Do you think you just eat too much, as you simply adore food, and that you have no restraint?

9 Do you tend to turn to food when you're bored, tired, unhappy or stressed?

10 Do you measure how well you have done each day by how little you have eaten and if you have managed to skip a meal?

11 Does food equal guilt?

As you have probably discovered after working through the above lists, an event in your past may have affected how you relate to food and eating. Food then begins to control you, sometimes so insidiously that you don't even recognise what is happening – and then it takes over your life.

There are many emotional triggers, including the need for comfort, rebellion, anxiety, sadness or escape, which cause you to eat in that 'out of control' way.

Chemicals in the brain, called neurotransmitters, are linked to mood and hunger, and they are responsible for carrying messages around the body. So, as food is associated with our first emotional trigger, it is not surprising that if, say, you feel intense emotions, you will simply think that food will make you feel better, happier or more comforted.

LIBERATE YOURSELF FROM ALL THIS

Hypnodiet will help you to identify the emotional triggers that cause you to eat when you are not hungry or to satisfy an emotion. It will assist you in developing new coping mechanisms to deal with the problem areas and delete them, so that you can begin to enjoy food as it becomes an ordinary part of your life.

Daily Hypnodiet meditations will not, of course, 'cure' you of an unhappy or painful past, or magically erase all life's stresses, but they will certainly help you to feel happier about yourself. Hypnodiet meditations allow you to bypass the complex associations and emotions that you have developed over the years with food. (I explain exactly how this works in Chapter 4.)

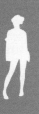

Hypnodiet is the key to ending a destructive relationship with food and to help you rediscover exercise.

If you are prepared to commit to Hypnodiet, you really can break the harmful cycle of overeating and dieting that you have become caught up in. Food can become a pleasure again – something you need, something you will enjoy but are not psychologically dependent upon. It really is that simple.

Getting back into the exercise habit

When you feel overweight and unattractive, exercise is the last thing you feel like doing, but that is exactly what makes us feel better about ourselves and helps us to look and feel good every day. Exercise is an essential part of your everyday life and not an optional extra. It is a key to reaching and maintaining a healthy size and weight. And when you exercise, you actually feel like eating less.

According to the British Nutrition Foundation, studies show that we usually don't eat more to make up for the energy we used when exercising. You probably know all too well that if you try to cut out 500 calories a day, you will feel very hungry. But if you burn off an extra 500 calories a day through exercise, you probably won't notice yourself feeling more hungry than usual. It really does make sense to move more! It's that wonderful balance of calories in and calories out that helps you to achieve a healthy weight. Hypnodiet will make you want to rediscover exercise again.

Chapter 3

WHAT'S NORMAL?

With Hypnodiet, you will be able to reprogramme your mind so that you develop a normal and healthy relationship with food. But to do this, first you have to understand what 'normal' is.

GETTING IN TOUCH

A 'normal' relationship with food is one that is free from guilt, self-punishment and emotional triggers. When you eat normally you savour your food: you really do enjoy eating. But you are not obsessed with food. You are in touch with

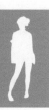

When you eat normally, you listen to your body and its basic needs.

your body. You choose foods that your body needs to stay healthy and fit for life. You might sometimes really want a square of chocolate. That's fine. But equally, sometimes you might really crave an apple or some steamed broccoli.

Normal eating means:

1 You will want to eat when your body needs to eat.

2 You will desire foods that your body needs and wants at that time.

3 You will want to stop when your body has had enough: you'll feel full, and eating won't be appealing any more.

4 Food will simply be food – a delicious source of sustenance. It will not be a punishment or a reward, or a guilty pleasure or a destructive act. It's just food.

HOW TO ENJOY YOUR FOOD

Most people eat while they are doing other things. They gobble breakfast while reading the paper or running for the tube train. At lunch, they shovel down a sandwich at their desk, or gulp it on the run between meetings. Dinner happens in front of the TV, or surrounded by chat and the hubbub of friends or family. There is virtually no time to enjoy the food, to think about the act of eating – to savour it.

★ **Case Study:** Lucy

LUCY, A 41-YEAR-OLD writer and mother of three, described how easy it is to eat without thinking about it – what I call 'mindless eating':

'I eat my breakfast while talking to my kids, getting up and down from the table, running all over the place – I hardly notice the toast go down. I snack in the mornings as I check my emails or do some work. I'll then eat my lunch over the newspaper, with the radio on, sometimes while talking on the phone. I snack in the afternoon as I prepare food for my children. I'll then eat the evening meal while talking to my children or husband, with music or the radio on in the background . . . I literally never just eat. I barely notice the taste of my food; what goes in, how much (unless to feel guilty!). And yet I'll tell anyone that I absolutely love eating.'

PUT THE BRAKES ON

I have lost count of the number of people who have told me that they adore food. Most of them eat very fast. They barely give themselves time to taste their food, let alone adore it. I always tell them, 'If you enjoy your food so much, why not slow down and get even more pleasure out of eating?'

I teach my clients to pay attention to what they are putting in their mouths; to think about how the food makes them feel, physically and emotionally. This is a far more pleasurable, satisfying and healthy way to eat. Eating this way will help you to consume only what your body needs – no more and no less. This is what I mean by 'mindful eating'.

WHAT IS MINDFULNESS?

Mindfulness is a psychological discipline with its origins in Buddhism. It is becoming increasingly popular as people search for a more serene and thoughtful way to live in our hectic modern world. Mindfulness techniques are also now used by mainstream psychologists to tackle issues such as chronic pain, cancer survival or depression. It is proven by numerous studies to be a clinically useful tool.

When it comes to eating healthily, the mindful approach can be enormously helpful. If you eat mindfully – that is, give eating your full attention – you will enjoy your food far more than you do now. You won't rush through meals. You will eat calmly. You will find it easy not to overeat.

So, how do you do it? Well, it's incredibly simple – although it may require some planning, and it will probably mean breaking some long-held bad habits.

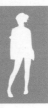

When you eat mindfully, eating will become a genuine pleasure.

How to eat mindfully

1 **Give eating your full attention**. Switch off the TV, the radio; put aside that newspaper or book. It is important to carve out a calm, quiet time for eating, where you are sitting down at a table and giving your full attention to your meal.

2 **Really appreciate your food**: arrange your food attractively on the plate and not haphazardly piled high in a mess. Take in the colours, textures and the aromas before you eat it – enjoy how beautiful food can be.

3 **Really taste your food**: when you put the food into your mouth appreciate the tastes and textures on your tongue; enjoy the different flavours. Paying attention like this will make each bite a choice rather than a reflex or a habit.

4 **Chew your food** – chew each mouthful 10 or 12 times. It's astonishing how fast most of us eat. Mindful eating will make you more aware of how much and how fast you usually eat. When you slow down, and chew and savour your food, you can tune into your body – when your brain sends the signal that you've had enough, you will listen.

5 **Think about how you feel as you eat**. Ask yourself if you like the taste of the food you're choosing right now? How do you feel as you eat? Happy? Excited? Anxious? Optimistic? Sad? Try not to judge the feeling, and don't try to change it. Simply observe it happening to you. Be curious about how eating makes you feel.

SAY GOODBYE TO EATING WITHOUT ENJOYMENT

It really is straightforward. And it is also surprisingly liberating – not to mention enjoyable! If you break the habit of
mindless eating – of gobbling your food without thought or,
indeed, much real pleasure – then you will get back in touch
with the process of eating. You will find that you can now
listen to your body. You will know when you feel satisfied
and have had enough to eat, so you won't want to eat any
more. This, in a nutshell, is 'normal' eating.

LOSING THE GUILT

It is not 'normal' to feel guilty every time you have something
to eat which you would not consider to be healthy. Occasional
treats – a few squares of chocolate, a small slice of cake – are
delicious. They are also a perfectly normal – if small – part of
any balanced diet. Normal eaters *do* occasionally have a treat!

★ **Case Study:** Andy

ANDY, A BANKER IN HIS FIFTIES, found that his weight had
been creeping up steadily over the years thanks to
frequently 'wining and dining' his clients. Hypnodiet
helped Andy to make healthy choices – even when eating
out. Eating mindfully also helped him to eat much
smaller portions of food. If you are eating more slowly, the
temptation to guzzle down huge portions is minimised.

Andy quickly and painlessly lost the weight. He felt fantastic, energised and rejuvenated – he even took up squash. At our final session, he described to me how Hypnodiet helped him to lose the guilt he used to feel around food:

'Yesterday I had a hunger day where I did want a small piece of cake. Then I remembered that you had said, "It is OK to have treats . . . that's normal," so, instead of feeling guilty, I had the piece of cake, and I enjoyed it to the full. I did think of you as I was eating it and I smiled to myself.'

HypnoDIET tip

Eat breakfast

It is normal to have breakfast, it is *essential* to have breakfast. Many people skip this meal, believing that it's not really necessary, and that by skipping it they will cut some calories. It is also the easiest meal to skip if you're rushing.

However, skipping breakfast is likely to backfire. If you skip breakfast, your blood-sugar levels will be too low. You will therefore begin to crave sugary, fatty boosts. It is then easy to get into the blood sugar 'surge-and-crash' cycle: you crave that mid-morning doughnut and coffee; it gives you an energy boost, but soon afterwards you get another sugar crash; you then crave a second doughnut, or a chocolate biscuit, or something equally energy dense. Your body is telling you it needs energy.

A HEALTHY BREAKFAST IS THE BEST START

Eating a substantial, healthy breakfast – something like a bowl of porridge with skimmed milk, plus chopped fruit and nuts – will avoid this surge-and-crash cycle. A good breakfast will fill you up. It will also regulate your blood-sugar levels, releasing energy slowly. You will therefore feel less 'desperate' later, and your body will not 'crave' unhealthy snacks.

GREAT BREAKFAST IDEAS

A good breakfast, ideally, should be a 'balanced meal' in its own right. As the saying goes, you should 'breakfast like a king'. This means, essentially, trying to include some whole-grain carbohydrate (such as porridge oats or wholemeal toast), some good fat (such as nuts or seeds), some fruit or vegetable and some protein (milk, egg, kippers, lean grilled bacon or ham) in your breakfast whenever you can. Here are three ideas:

1   Porridge made with skimmed milk. Add a handful of chopped nuts and some blueberries.
2   Scrambled egg on wholemeal toast with a tomato or a piece of fruit.
3   A slice of ham or cheese on a wholegrain bagel with a piece of fruit or a tomato on the side.

GETTING THE PORTIONS RIGHT

If you want to learn how to eat healthily, it really is important to establish what a sensible portion size should be. Research shows that when we're served a larger portion we tend to eat it all; so, not only do we eat more than we would have but we also feel that we *should* eat it all, because it's on our plate. However, when we've eaten it that larger portion doesn't necessarily make us feel any more satisfied.

DOWNSIZING

In today's supersize culture it's all too easy to get into the habit of eating much more than you need. Portion sizes in restaurants and takeaways are getting bigger all the time and it is indicative that more and more restaurants are providing 'doggy bags' to take home: we just can't finish the portions that are being served. This doesn't make sense to me at all, and I can't understand why the restaurant owners don't think, 'Perhaps our portions sizes are too big!' One study by the World Cancer Research Fund found that burgers have doubled in size since 1980 and pasta servings are about five times larger.

So here's a brief portion guide. Please don't become obsessive about portions, or start weighing food, simply be aware that a sensible portion is probably *way* smaller than your usual one. It's time to readjust.

Sensible portion sizes

- Dried pasta – a small tea cup
- Dried rice – a small tea cup
- Cereal – one third of a cereal bowl, but you can have half a bowlful of cooked porridge oats
- Cheese – two slithers just for the taste
- Fish – one small salmon steak, or lemon sole or plaice, and so on
- Meat – a small chicken breast or equivalent amount of meat
- Nuts – a small handful is a good snack size

Portion tips

- Use a smaller plate.
- Serve yourself lots of vegetables, especially greens (but limit potatoes). You can have half a plateful of mixed vegetables such as broccoli, tomatoes, peppers, courgettes, green beans, peas, lettuce and mushrooms.
- Cook less food, then you won't be tempted to eat large portions or second helpings.
- Don't eat from the packet: put a sensible portion into a bowl so that you can see how much you're eating.
- At a party, take one small portion of the various nibbles and eat them from a side plate rather than constantly scooping up handfuls from the large serving bowls.

GIVE YOUR BRAIN A CHANCE

It takes up to 20 minutes for your brain to register that your stomach is full and to let you know that you have had enough to eat. If you eat quickly and continue eating until you simply can't eat any more, or if you take second helpings or determinedly finish your supersize portion, you won't know whether you are full or not until it's too late – when you've eaten way more than you need!

HypnoDIET tip
How to normalise your eating

'Normal' eating is about understanding that the impulse to reach for a muffin could well stem from an emotional, and not a physical, need. Normal eating means that you only eat when you are genuinely hungry. You don't eat to heal past or present hurts, to fill emotional voids, to comfort or entertain yourself. You eat because you are hungry. And you eat moderate amounts – you don't binge or starve yourself – and you always stop when you have had enough.

When you eat normally, no food is 'sinful' – there is no guilt, no self-denial or obsession. Instead, you pay attention to what your body needs and when it needs it. You nurture yourself by choosing healthy, life-enhancing foods, and yes, having the odd treat as well. Once you begin to eat normally, you will experience a huge sense of liberation. Life truly can become significantly less complicated – and it can start today.

It's vital to put small and sensible portions onto your plate, to eat slowly and to wait and be more mindful before you reach for second helpings.

Keep active

Remember that exercise is essential to keeping your body trim and your mind happy. You'll find that when you exercise you will eat less, so it really does need to be part of every day of your life, as I explain in Chapter 7.

KEEP A FOOD DIARY

A food diary can be a good tool for anyone who wants to lose weight and establish a more 'mindful' attitude to food. I encourage my clients to write down what they eat and drink each day – everything they consume. I ask them to note down what time it is when they eat – as this shows how regular their eating patterns are – how early in the day they start eating and how late in the day they finish. Doing this can give you a valuable insight: are you a 'grazer' (you eat constantly throughout the day) or do you skip meals?

I also ask clients to note down their physical activity – what kind of activity, how long for, and when.

Finally, next to each meal, I ask them to write down how they felt at the time, because emotions can trigger eating binges. Do they feel tired for no apparent reason or have a bloated stomach? This can indicate food intolerances.

THE BIGGER PICTURE

Keeping a food diary like this will help you to build up a picture of what you are eating, when and why. It will help you to work out how best to fit exercise into your day, and to notice how exercise affects the way you eat.

Sometimes, it is only when we see it in black and white on the page that we begin to understand not just what 'triggers' us to eat but also what encourages us to eat well.

WHAT A DIARY TELLS US

Alan's diary, overleaf, shows a cycle of mounting pressure, work-related stress and tiredness – all of which have an impact on Alan's eating patterns. He feels tired and fuels himself with sugar in a sugar-rush–sugar-crash cycle throughout the day. He relies on black coffee to wake him up or keep him going, and, in stress, he turns to sugary snacks for comfort and energy.

Alan is so busy he finds himself caught short when hungry, so reaches for the closest thing: peanuts and chocolate on the train, the pizza delivery at the end of the day. His lifestyle and lack of planning mean that he is constantly rushing, feeling guilty and tired. He manages only four glasses of water in the whole day (aim for eight if you can!). His diet is very low in fruit and vegetables, and he tends to eat them, not because he wants to but rather as an afterthought because he feels guilty.

How a food diary works

Alan, aged 52, is a PR executive. This is his first food diary:

7.00 a.m. 1 glass of water. Feeling really tired.
Dreading long day ahead. Black coffee.

8.30 a.m. Brisk walk 10 mins from tube to office.
Still tired, anxious about big meeting.
1 double espresso coffee, blueberry muffin.
Perk up.

11.00 a.m. Starving and tired again. Deadlines add
pressure. 2 chocolate biscuits.
Black coffee.

1.00 p.m. Business lunch: fillet of salmon, 6 roast
potatoes, green beans in butter,
bread roll and butter. Feel stressed – rush to
eat lunch. To-do list at back of mind.
1 large glass of wine, 2 glasses of sparkling
water.

4.00 p.m. Stressed and tired. 2 chocolate biscuits and
black coffee.

7.30 p.m. Exhausted. Anxious about work. 1 bag of
roasted peanuts and chocolate bar on the
train. Guilt – five a day? Apple.

8.30 p.m. Pepperoni pizza delivered, three large glasses
of red wine. Feel better. Know I should eat
healthily but nothing in fridge and had a
hard day, so deserve it.

10.00 p.m. 1 glass of water before bed. Feel guilty about pizza and wine, must do better tomorrow. Exhausted. Anxious about tomorrow. 2 chocolate biscuits.

A DIARY CAN HELP YOU MAKE SUCCESSFUL CHANGES

By keeping a diary like this, Alan was able to identify patterns of behaviour and how they affect his eating. Using Hypnodiet, he began to plan his meals and take healthy snacks with him to work. He began to feel happier, under less pressure and less anxious at work. He was able to feel more energised by cutting out the sugary snacks, and cutting down dramatically on the black coffee (he still drinks coffee but now mostly decaffeinated).

Alan drinks much more water these days and is nearer to achieving his goal of 'five a day'. He says he has amazed himself at how much more energy he has. He has more free time and even found time to exercise and to realise the benefits of doing so.

BE HONEST, FEEL BETTER

A food diary also allows you to be honest about how much you are eating. This, surprisingly, can actually stop you from tormenting yourself. Often, people feel as if they are eating huge amounts, but when they write down exactly what they do eat, they see that it's really not that bad. This, in turn, cuts down on the self-sabotaging thoughts: *Well, I've blown it already today – I might as well pig out on this dinner!*

Keeping a food diary really is worth the small amount of effort.

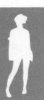

Studies have shown that a food diary is a valuable tool that can help aid weight loss.

Start your food diary today

I recommend buying a small, pocket-sized notebook and keeping this with you at all times. Note down what you've eaten and how you feel straight away, rather than going back over the day. It takes only a few seconds but it will really help you to build an honest picture of your lifestyle and emotions. Also, remember to write down any exercise.

YOU *CAN* GET OUT OF THAT HOLE

Most people who come to me believe that their problems with food are so deep-seated, go so far back, and are so profound that they will never be sorted out in just a session or two, but this is simply not true.

Hypnodiet can help you to bypass the emotional associations you have with food (I explain exactly how this works in Chapter 7). Best of all, you can feel it working almost immediately.

★ **Case Study:** Leyla

LEYLA, THE PAEDIATRICIAN CLIENT I introduced earlier, told me:

'I did feel much calmer and more positive after our session. Straight away I noticed that I was far more patient at work, and also with my own kids at home. I wasn't shouting and I did feel happier. On the second week, I went out for dinner with my husband and some friends, and as we walked into the restaurant, music was playing and I started to dance and sing and to laugh. It felt really good. I thought, Wow, I'm really enjoying myself!

'Later on, it made me cry to realise how sad my life had become, but then I thought about the things you had said: how it is time to learn to love myself and to rediscover my sensuality; how all that is part of Hypnodiet. I've been eating so much better now – it really does feel more "normal". I'm eating slowly, keeping my food diary and leaving food on my plate. I feel like I'm beginning to love life again and to love myself.'

> *With Hypnodiet you will no longer worry or constantly think about eating.*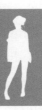

You will find that as you start Hypnodiet, your food obsessions will fade away. You will eat when you are hungry, but the panic and urgency will vanish.

★ **Case Study:** Derek

DEREK told me in his second session:

'I was amazed at how quickly I became relaxed about eating. It was like being released from a kind of prison – I had a huge sense of freedom.'

As soon as you've had your first Hypnodiet meditation, you will begin to feel the changes in your behaviour and attitude straight away. The effects are instant, sometimes dramatic and sometimes subtle; that's the beauty of hypnosis. As you continue with Hypnodiet, you will see many more changes over the coming weeks and months.

Chapter 4

RELAX – THE MYTHS AND FEARS SURROUNDING HYPNOSIS

P eople often ask me how hypnosis works. I tell them that it's a relatively simple, fast and straightforward tool that changes your behaviour from the inside out. But how exactly does it do this?

THE ASTONISHING POWER OF THE MIND

Hypnosis is defined as a state of deep relaxation within your body and a state of increased and heightened awareness within your mind. However, for years hypnosis has caused intrigue and still does to this day, but the misconception that hypnosis 'messes with your mind' and you will never be the same again is simply not true. It is popularly believed that hypnosis is a state resembling sleep and almost of unconsciousness, but scientific research has proven time and time again that hypnosis is actually a wakeful state of focused attention and heightened awareness and suggestibility.

Hypnosis allows you to access your creative potential. This is how all those long-held thoughts, beliefs and patterns of behaviour can be deleted and rewritten. It isn't magic, it's the astonishing power of the mind.

Note

JUST TO AVOID CONFUSION, HYPNOTHERAPY IS SIMPLY HYPNOSIS BEING USED FOR THERAPEUTIC REASONS, AND IS THEREFORE REFERRED TO AS HYPNOTHERAPY.

★ **Case Study:** Sylvia

WHEN I FIRST SAW SYLVIA, a TV producer in her thirties, she was a size 16 and she had battled with her weight since early adolescence. Her pattern was to binge on food and alcohol, then purge with strict diets and detox regimes. She lost and gained a lot of weight, but over the years the scales crept up until she felt she was completely out of control.

Sylvia wanted to be a size 10 and to liberate herself

from the pain and stress of all these years of fearful dieting. She achieved her target after five months. When I saw her for our final session she looked like a different person: glowing, happy and confident. As we talked, after the session, she said to me:

'I don't know what you have done, but it's as though you have somehow short-circuited my system.'

DELETING NEGATIVE THOUGHTS

Sylvia had put her finger right on it: hypnosis does work by short-circuiting – or deleting – negative patterns of thought or behaviour, and in a short period of time. Hypnodiet allowed Sylvia to short-circuit all those negative, self-hating thoughts – the messages she'd absorbed over the years from her critical mother, from her friends or acquaintances, or from the media, that she was somehow less worthwhile if she was overweight, less loved, less desirable – less 'legitimate'.

Hypnodiet, of course, is not a 'cure' for years of unhappiness or abuse, and it won't change our culture. It is simply a way to bypass all those unhelpful thoughts and impulses, replacing

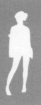

Hypnosis is one of the most powerful states for personal development and positive change.

them with new, healthy patterns of behaviour. Through deep
relaxation, and reprogramming the mind, using her daily meditations and visualisations, Sylvia was able to short-circuit the
years of bad eating habits and low self-esteem. The process felt,
she told me, like 'a miracle'.

> *Hypnodiet will replace your*
> *unhealthy eating patterns with*
> *new and healthy ones.*

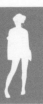

DOES IT WORK FOR EVERYBODY?

You, of course, may be thinking, *It will never happen
that way for me*. Well, the first thing to understand
about hypnosis is that virtually everybody has their doubts
about whether it will work for them – or indeed, for
anyone!

★ **Case Study:** Sylvia

SYLVIA admitted to me in her final session:

'*I did have doubts. I've sometimes thought to myself, Is it
going to work? It feels almost too good to be true that I
will never have a weight issue again. But then I look at
myself and I realise that it has worked. It is simply
amazing.*'

Practice makes perfect

Hypnosis only works if you practise, in order to reinforce the messages. So, remember that you need to listen to the CD every day until you have reached your target size. Then, to keep the message in the forefront of your mind, listen to the meditations twice a week to maintain the new you.

HOW HYPNOSIS WORKS

I began my career as a psychologist, but was drawn to hypnotherapy because I realised that hypnosis could bring about far quicker, longer-lasting results. I am aware of just how powerful the mind can be, and the combination of results plus speed fascinated me. When you are on a diet it takes days to see results, unless you use one of the many drastic diets and starve yourself (although that weight usually comes back later). Hypnosis, however, is instant, because the effects are seen from the moment you open your eyes – and it is all natural. It's an amazing tool for change.

Of course, not all hypnotherapy – or hypnotherapists, for that matter – are the same, and many have different ways of working. Some are therefore more effective than others, but the basic principles are the same. To describe how hypnosis works, it is often easiest to turn first to the four most common misconceptions about it.

MYTH 1: I WILL BE 'PUT UNDER'

Many people think that when they are hypnotised, they will somehow lose consciousness – become zombielike and unable to control their actions. They also think that afterwards they might forget what happened – that the session will be a total blank. These are very popular beliefs, but they are wrong.

FACT With hypnosis generally – and certainly the kind I practice – you do not hand over your control (or your dignity!) to me. The state of deep relaxation that you reach during hypnosis is known as REM (rapid eye movement) or the 'dream state' – a term you may have heard used for describing sleep patterns.

Hypnosis resembles the state you are in as you enter sleep: you are not fully asleep but you are not fully awake either, just very deeply relaxed. Because the body has slowed down, REM automatically takes place. (It is worth noting that REM takes place during the lightest part of your sleeping state and that you can easily be woken from this state; it is the state where the dreaming takes place. So, if you are woken during REM sleep, you will invariably remember your dream.) You get into that state purely by relaxing your body and mind, guided by my voice and my instructions. With Hypnodiet, you can do this at home, using the CD.

In this relaxed, guided state you will be calm but alert –
more hyper-attentive than drowsy. You 'tune out' from
everything around you but remain alert and focused. You
can get up and walk away at any time during a hypnotherapy session. You can choose to ignore or blot out the whole
thing; or you can choose to let it in.

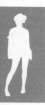

*Hypnosis is almost like losing
yourself in an amazing book.*

In other words, hypnosis is not something that's done *to*
you – it's something you do *for yourself*. It stands to reason,
therefore, that the more motivated you are the better
Hypnodiet will work for you.

MYTH 2: SOME PEOPLE CAN'T BE HYPNOTISED

Most people, during their first session, think 'it's not working'. They feel wide awake, fully conscious – even critical –
and assume that this means they are in some way resistant to
the method (or that the hypnotherapist is having an off day!).

FACT Some people are certainly easier to hypnotise than
others, but virtually anybody can be hypnotised very effec-
tively by a hypnotherapist who knows what he or she is doing.

MYTH 3: IT'S ALL MUMBO-JUMBO

People often think, *Well, there's no scientific proof to show that hypnosis works, so why should I believe it? It can't possibly work; after all, it's just some stranger telling me to behave in a certain way. Why would I take any notice of that?*

FACT It is certainly true that science has yet to come up with a definitive and watertight explanation for exactly how hypnosis works. But then, there is a lot that science does not yet understand about the workings of the human mind. Essentially, it is clear that when you are under hypnosis you are in a more 'suggestible' state. Scientific studies using electroencephalographs have found that under hypnosis the activity of the brain changes – it begins to show more sleeplike patterns than conscious, waking ones. And yet you feel lucid. In other words, it seems that during hypnosis the conscious mind – with all its doubts, fears and anxieties – takes a back seat. This allows the subconscious mind to open up.

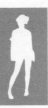

I will access your subconscious mind to help you to change your attitude to food.

The subconscious mind is responsible not just for your impulses and emotions but for your creativity and imagination too. As your hypnotherapist, I will delete unhelpful 'files' from your subconscious and replace them with helpful ones that you will then act upon, even when your conscious mind takes over (I'll explain this further in Chapter 5).

MYTH 4: HYPNOSIS DOESN'T WORK

Some people find it difficult to believe that a person can change their behaviour, or cope with pain, simply by relaxing and listening while someone speaks to them in a quiet and peaceful way, and they feel certain that hypnosis couldn't possibly work for them.

FACT During my 23 years as a hypnotherapist I have seen countless people conquer their weight and eating problems (not to mention other issues, such as alcohol or drug dependency) using hypnotherapy. Countless women have used hypnosis techniques to cope with the pain and anxiety of childbirth. Many others use hypnosis to help with undergoing dental work, or to tackle phobias. It has worked for them and it can work for you too.

But you don't have to take my word for this. There are numerous well-documented cases of hypnosis being used as the only form of anaesthesia for surgery, including gall-bladder removal, amputation, caesarean section and hysterectomy. Hypnosis is used in medical settings around the world to help people cope with anything from cancer to allergies, gastrointestinal problems, chronic pain, burns and hypertension (high blood pressure).

It is also, of course, a well-established tool in mainstream psychotherapy, helping people to tackle issues such as anxiety or sleep disorders.

HypnoDIET tip
Background noise

It is always best to do your meditations when you are unlikely to be disturbed. Switch off your phones and shut the door. But this is the real world too, so you may hear noises coming from another room or outside while you are listening to the CD. These will not disturb you. It is normal to be aware of your surroundings during hypnosis. The difference is that you will feel incredibly relaxed and free from tension. Even with some background noise, you can reach a state of peace and tranquillity.

Hypnosis is a state of mind

It may surprise you to learn that you can hypnotise yourself successfully. The only requirements for success are for you to achieve a relaxed state where the mind is more open and for you to be willing to take suggestions as you listen to my voice. (Incidentally, the monotonous tone of my voice and repeated suggestions are deliberate and necessary, as this induces a sleep-like trance so that you become totally relaxed. I am therefore able to instil the required changes into your subconscious mind.)

During the process of self-hypnosis I will teach you to first remove the negative patterns of thought and behaviour, which created failure in the first place, and then to reprogramme your mind for success with the new beliefs necessary to make the desired changes.

Self-hypnosis

For Hypnodiet to work you need only to be in a light state of hypnosis. It is perfectly possible to put yourself into this state. We are all in a state of hypnosis at certain times during the day, whether we realise this or not. Many would say it was just daydreaming, but it is often a mild hypnotic state – in effect, self-hypnosis.

MOTIVATION

Hypnodiet is a tool that will help anyone who has decided for themselves – rather than being pressurised by a critical friend, partner or parent – that they would like to lose weight. If you think you're fine the way you are, but are only doing this because your partner says you are fat, you may well struggle with Hypnodiet.

The good thing is, though, that anybody who is truly motivated can use Hypnodiet to slim down and develop a normal, healthy relationship with food for the rest of their life.

It is, then, a total myth that you have to be on a diet in order to lose weight and get to your ideal size.

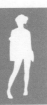

This is something you have to do for yourself – but I will help you.

★ **Case Study:** Sylvia

SYLVIA also told me the last time I treated her:

'I've surprised myself at how much better I have been, I haven't been eating between meals and haven't even thought about doing so. The other day there were lots of goodies around the office, and someone's birthday

cupcakes, and I have never, ever refused them before. I just didn't want them. It was quite a revelation. I absolutely love it!'

But, once again, don't take my word for it – or Sylvia's. You can discover the power of hypnosis for yourself. It's all up to you.

Chapter 5

YOUR DELETE BUTTON

Believe it or not, there was once a time when eating, for you, was straightforward. There was no anxiety, guilt or stress. You just ate because you were hungry and stopped eating because you were full. But why did this change?

THE COMFORT OF FOOD

Many people have had experiences that have made them turn to food for comfort. It's not surprising really. The urge to comfort eat is instinctive. As babies, our cries were comforted by cuddles and our mother's milk; as children there were treats if we hurt ourselves, or rewards when we behaved well. As adults, that same urge can easily be triggered. There are countless reasons why people comfort eat: anxiety, stress or any number of challenging life events, such as divorce, bereavement, emotional or physical trauma. People comfort eat to get themselves through relationship problems, or to counter the feeling that they are unloved. A lack of self-confidence, insecurity or low self-esteem can also make us turn to food. Sometimes, we simply eat to stave off boredom, cheer ourselves up or reward ourselves after a hard day.

BREAKING FREE

Hypnodiet enables you to break the connection between difficult emotions and food. You'll still feel the emotion, but it won't lead you straight to the biscuit tin. The impulse to snack may be there sometimes, but the connection will not be made.

Using the meditations on the CD, I am going to help you to find the moment when your relationship with food changed. I will enable you to locate this moment, and then, quite literally, help you to 'delete' that moment from your subconscious mind.

You've broken the deep-seated connections that lead you to overeat, and, from now on, you will eat normally and healthily. Eating will no longer be fraught, guilt-ridden or obsessive. Food is just food – you've deleted the rest.

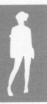

Once you've found that delete button, and pressed it, you can move on: you're free!

ONE STEP TO A NEW LIFE

By pressing your delete button it is possible to erase any emotional complexities that cause you to eat in an unhealthy way. You can then move forward into a new and straightforward relationship with food and exercise that will stay with you for life.

I know this sounds unlikely, but it really does work. I've seen it happen in countless people – even those whose lives were painful and complicated, and whose eating problems go back many years.

LOCATING THE PAINFUL EXPERIENCE

Everybody who is eating too much and is overweight has encountered something that has caused the problem, and the first step towards recovery is to locate the experience. This is where the 'delete button' will lie. As a hypnotherapist I have heard all kinds of stories from people who are held in the clutches of a bad relationship with food. Here are some of them.

★ **Case Study:** Carly

CARLY, 40, A TV PRODUCER, had struggled with her weight for decades before she came to see me.

'*I am bored with myself and all this bingeing, food and alcohol. My mum has a weight problem and all my teenage and adult life I have been involved with diets one way or another. I remember that when my mum was on one of her diets, biscuits and cakes would be banned from the house. It seemed so unfair at the time that I shouldn't be allowed these things just because she was on a diet. Even now I feel the same sense of injustice when I try to deprive myself of food. So I rebel and eat even more.'*

Carly can identify exactly when her relationship with food switched from simply feeding the body, to feeding an emotional need as well:

'One day I overheard my mum say she could not cope with me and that she wished she had never had children. Before that I never had a weight problem, but after that, I just seemed to eat and eat.'

Carly was now eating, not to satisfy hunger, but for comfort and reassurance, to make herself feel loved, and to cope with anxiety. Over the years, her weight slowly escalated.

'My mum told me last year that I am an embarrassment to her and I just cried – on my own of course, I never let anyone see me cry. I never let anybody see me eat a lot of food either – I do that in secret too.'

And then, she began to sob uncontrollably – opening up for the first time about her years of pain and secrecy.

EMOTIONAL SENSITIVITY WHEN OUR
BODIES CHANGE

Sometimes the delete button lies in adolescence, and some people find that their eating habits are tied up with their sexuality.

Adolescence is a particularly sensitive time. A time when your sense of self is just developing, your hormones and emotions are all over the place and you are exploring who you are. This is also the time when you are building up self-esteem and a sense of your own competence and security. If you are told that you are inadequate, or if traumatic things happen to you, the emotional impact can last a lifetime.

You may be uncomfortable with the changes in your body during adolescence. Girls develop rounded, shapely areas, which they can feel embarrassed about, especially if siblings or parents notice and comment. Those comments can make them feel overweight, so that they turn to food for comfort or self-punishment – or both.

These patterns, created by difficult emotions 'solved' (or

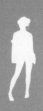

Hypnodiet will break harmful patterns caused by difficult emotions and will free you to develop and to enjoy your adolescence and adulthood.

worsened) by food, can be hard to break and can stay with you for life.

FEELING TOO SELF-CONSCIOUS

Some women continue to feel uncomfortable about their bodies into adulthood when they receive attention from men.

★ **Case Study:** Anna

ANNA, 30, AN 'OUT OF WORK' ACTRESS, was an unhappy size 20 when she came to me. She had been overweight as a teenager, became very slim in her early twenties, and then gained a lot of weight, very quickly.

'I hate being addicted to food and I hate being fat. But I also hate the attention I got from men when I was a size 10. I just couldn't handle it – I had never had this attention before in my life. I couldn't cope with men being so predatory and flirtatious.'

In other words, Anna's weight gain was in part a self-protection mechanism.

MORE THAN JUST A MOMENT

Of course, it's often not as simple as identifying an instant where everything changed, or to find a reason for it. Indeed, it can sometimes feel that the 'moment' when your eating changed is actually way more than a moment – it's an entire period of your life.

★ **Case Study:** Alice

ALICE, 22, came to see me last year. An immensely private, almost suspicious person, she was obviously very unhappy with her life. At a size 12/14, she felt that food was controlling her (her target was a size 10). She had been on diets since she was 12 years old, but her issues with food stretched further back than this.

Alice's childhood was miserable. Her parents – a model and a 'failed singer in a rock-and-roll band' – separated when she was a baby. She has two older sisters, both with similar weight issues. The three girls were raised by their mother – an alcoholic and cocaine addict. *'I remember when I was ten years old I came home from school and my mum was in a state. She was afraid to be left on her own, so I had to look after her. I was scared too.*

'My mum just partied and partied and never spent time with me. I loved her, but she didn't seem to love me. She said I was annoying. I think I found comfort in food from a very early age. She told me once that I was very resourceful as a baby. When I was about 18 months old she could go out all night partying; if she didn't get back until the morning, she said, I'd be OK because she left me food at the bottom of my cot and a bottle of milk in case I woke up.'

At this point in our session Alice broke down, unable to continue for a short while. It turned out that Alice's father, too, had been absent.

'My dad was hardly ever around. On the rare occasions when he took me out in his amazing cars, he loved me to open the glove box, and chocolates would fall out – there were so many . . . and they were all for me. I would take some of the chocolates to give to my friends at school, but mostly I'd hide them under the bed and eat them myself in private.'

In other words, food became a stand-in for the love and stability she so badly craved. It became a source of comfort and reassurance through the turmoil of her childhood. The result is that Alice cannot eat normally. 'I hate my body and have no self-esteem or confidence at all. I wish I had died when I tried to kill myself, then I wouldn't be a burden to anyone and I wouldn't have to struggle with my weight.'

Alice's story shows that often a problem around food can be triggered not just by a moment or an incident but by an entire period of your life: your early childhood perhaps, a

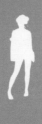

Hypnodiet works just as well whether your eating issues originate over a short or a long period of your life – and whether you can consciously identify an event or not.

difficult adolescence, or even a bad relationship that went on for years. This does not mean that you are 'incurable' and doomed to overeat for life.

MY APPROACH IS PERSONAL TO YOU

I am not here to psychoanalyse people like Alice, although many of my clients have similarly distressing stories, which I must admit I find very moving and they bring me to tears. While I was writing this book, I read aloud to myself so that I could put myself into the reader's shoes and feel what you may be feeling. As I read through, I felt, once again, the emotions of the day I encountered Alice, Anna and Carly, or the many I see every day in my consulting rooms in Harley Street or elsewhere in the world.

I am immensely passionate about my work and I want this passion to come through to you, so that you feel that I want to, and will, help you in the same sincere way that I have helped my other clients, whether you are in my consulting rooms or reading this book.

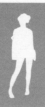

You are my personal client, and I want you to succeed and feel happy about yourself.

YOU *CAN* FIND THE ANSWER

Hypnodiet works with or without therapy, whether face to face or through reading my book and listening to the CD. It can help you to reach back to a time before these complexities began; a time in your life, possibly even as a tiny baby, when you ate to satisfy hunger, and nothing else. The desire for food is one of our first emotions.

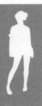

> *You can reach into your past and delete the subconscious memories that have caused you to overeat.*

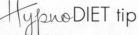 DIET tip

Exploring your past emotions

You may be apprehensive about exploring your past emotions, but there is no need to feel afraid. We all learn from our emotions. Learning is enlightening, and you will feel empowered as you take control of your eating and are able to enjoy just being you.

Of course, not everyone will be able to automatically pinpoint a 'moment' when it all changed. You may think that your childhood is far too complicated to pick through.

You may worry that your problems around food are so deep-seated that you'll never work out where it all started.

Equally, you may well think that your relationship with food is not complicated at all. You just love eating! People often say this to me, and I tell them that if they are consistently eating too much, then there is always some emotional attachment, however minor, that is preventing them from being their ideal size.

> **The good news**
>
> We all have a 'delete' button. We all have a time when food was simple and satisfying: a time when it was just food. Hypnodiet will help you find this time, and press that button.

HOW WILL YOU FIND YOUR OWN DELETE BUTTON?

Using the meditations on the CD, you will be able to reach a state of deep relaxation. It will then be possible to access either the moment when it all changed or the time when eating just felt natural to you. Don't worry, I will find that moment. Even though you may not be able to put your finger on the cause in your normal waking consciousness, the delete button *is* there and can be found during your meditations. What's more, you will find it during your first meditation. Here's how it works:

1   **Relax and go back.** As you listen to the accompanying CD you will enter a hypnotic state. I will then guide you to a place where, as a small baby being spoon-fed, you ate because you were hungry and you enjoyed the food. If you didn't like the taste of the food you just wouldn't eat it and no amount of coaxing from well-intentioned parents was going to persuade you. Also, at this time in your life, when you had eaten enough you would refuse to eat any more – you would turn your face away from the spoon, shut your mouth or shake your head. You instinctively knew how to express yourself, even though you couldn't speak yet.

2   **Find your turning point.** Then, when did that change? I will look for a transitional period in your life. When did you start to eat when you weren't hungry? When did you no longer need coaxing to eat more? When did you start to eat food that didn't taste good, but was just food – and at times, any food would do? I will help you to find that point through hypnosis on the CD, and then delete it.

3   **Keep the feeling.** I will then help you to bring the feeling when eating was just natural to you to the forefront of your mind.

4   **Press delete.** Finally, I will delete the emotional associations and complexities. Again, this is just like deleting files from a computer. These are defective files. You don't need them any more. I will help you to remove all the emotional associations that trigger your desire for food – whether they are comfort, boredom, stress or tiredness.

HypnoDIET tip

Let me do it for you

Don't worry! I'll do all the work. All you have to do is relax and follow the instructions. The beauty of Hypnodiet is that I will guide you through your past, but you will not find it anxiety provoking.

IT ALL HAPPENS IN YOUR SUBCONSCIOUS MIND

What's amazing about hypnosis is that you don't need to know, consciously, when your eating patterns changed in childhood.

Of course, I'm not saying that the emotions will just vanish into thin air. They are still in your subconscious somewhere. But the point is that once the connection is deleted, these emotions will no longer influence your eating habits. This is what I mean by pressing your delete button.

I CAN CHANGE YOUR MIND

Hypnosis is surrounded by mystery but it needn't be. Often a client will say to me, 'I don't know what you have done or how you do it, but it is as though you have somehow repro-grammed me to do the things I want to do and have been unable to. Yet I now do them without even trying.'

Many changes can be made though hypnosis and the power of the mind: I change your negative thoughts into positive ones. You may think you cannot achieve a task, such as having a normal healthy relationship with food, because you have been indoctrinated and weaned on that fact for years. Hypnosis enables those changes to happen.

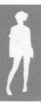

The mind is very powerful. You can change negatives into positives.

It's all learned behaviour

When a child is continually told they are clumsy, sure enough that child will grow into adulthood not so gracefully: stepping on people's toes, dropping things and bumping into people and objects – that is, until they are reprogrammed to believe that they are not clumsy at all. After all, they were not born clumsy, they have just learned to be, because they have been told continually that that is what they are.

Any learned behaviour is the same, such as eating disorders or simply unhealthy eating patterns; people are not born that way, they learned it.

WHAT HAPPENS NOW?

From now on, food will be a simple matter of pleasurable, healthy sustenance. You will eat because you're hungry, not because you need comfort or love, or you feel anxious. The delete button is a powerful tool. It's time to find yours and press it!

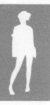

Pressing your delete button takes just a few minutes – but it can last a lifetime.

★ **Case Study:** Danni

FROM THE MOMENT DANNI, 38 and a PR executive, came to see me, she was on the defensive. She didn't really believe that I could help her. After all no one else had, so why should I be any different? She had come to me out of desperation. After we'd talked for a few minutes she began to relax. She told me later that she realised that I really wanted to help her, and that I was sincere and passionate about this. That's when she decided to open up. It turned out that the negative comments of loved ones were causing her self-destructive eating.

'*If I'm going out to dinner and I know I'm going to be bad I think to myself, I might as well be bad all day and have a chocolate bar for breakfast. My dad said to me the other day, "I'm disappointed in you, Danni, I thought you would be the pretty, slim one and your sister would be the fat one like your mum, but just look at the state of you, you're fatter than the pair of them." You have no idea how that made me feel. I try to deny that I'm fat sometimes, I act all jolly with my friends so they'll like me, I guess. But I know I am kidding myself. I know I desperately need to lose this weight, for myself – to move forward with my life.*'

After our first hypnosis session, Danni told me that she was amazed with the results:

'I realise I can do this. You helped me to find my delete button and I felt this instant shift inside me. It felt liberating to have pressed delete on all those years of guilty overeating. I feel as if I'm on a mission now. It is strange, but I already feel lighter.'

Danni says she steadily lost 25kg (4st/56lb) over the next eight months. She is now a healthy size 12.

KEEPING THE MESSAGE STRONG

Hypnosis is always effective, but practising reinforces the message. In a way, it's the same as with exercise: you would exercise intensively in the beginning until you are happy with your body tone, then you would exercise less frequently each week to maintain your toned body. If you stop exercising you will quickly turn to flab. Hypnodiet works on the same principle: daily meditations with the CD will reinforce the message, which then needs to be just 'topped up' once or twice each week to maintain your body in its new, healthy and trim shape.

Practising the meditations reinforces the message.

Chapter 6

SEE YOURSELF SLIM

So, you want to be thinner? You want to 'look good'. You want to 'feel better'. But what does this actually mean? How much thinner will you become? And what, exactly, do you really mean by 'looking good'? How much better do you want to feel?

It is vital to have a clear goal from the outset. It's actually no good saying, 'I just want to be thinner.' I want you to be far more specific than that. To do this, it is important to build a clear picture in your mind of what you will become when you use Hypnodiet. This is called 'visualisation' and it will become an important part of your daily meditations.

YOUR IDEA OF THE NEW YOU

To create an effective visualisation for yourself, you first have to work out exactly what weight loss means to you.

You need to produce a clear picture of what you will look like when you lose the weight. To do this, you need to develop your very own Visualisation Tool.

HOW TO CREATE YOUR VISUALISATION TOOL

Many people initially find this part of the programme difficult to get their heads around. But bear with me; I will explain that although it may sound crazy it really does help.

Every new diet offers hope, but then disappointment quickly follows. As each diet is ditched the expectation becomes less. So, although you would like to believe that Hypnodiet will work for you and live up to its reputation, you are probably somewhat sceptical if you have tried, perhaps, ten different diets. When I ask you to visualise yourself the size you really *want* to be, you would love to believe you could achieve it, but your hopes have been dashed too many times, so you will probably decide to imagine a size that you think is 'more realistic'. But I say, don't go for that 'realistic' size, be bold and go for your *dream size* – and don't be afraid to do so!

Here's how to start:

1   You may have a favourite photograph of yourself taken when you were the ideal size, or you may prefer to flip through a magazine to find an image of the perfect body size – a size you've dreamed of becoming and you know this will be your body shape.

2   Superimpose your face from a favourite photograph onto the image of that ideal body. If you're a computer whiz, you may have a better way of doing this that allows you to print out a more 'realistic' picture of your own face on this ideal body.

3   When you settle down for your meditations, keep this photograph or picture with you. This might sound ridiculous, but most people have very visual brains. It is enormously helpful to be able to 'see' what you are aiming for – to visualise your future self at the size you want to be; the size you will become.

★ **Case study:** Sarah

SARAH, 43, works for a bank. She was a classic comfort eater, but visualisations kept her working towards her goal. Her mother had issues around food and, from the age of eight, so did Sarah. She was teased at school and nicknamed 'fatso'. As an adult she tended to eat more when feeling lonely or stressed. In our first session she said: *'I'll just binge eat anything in sight. I can have chocolate, chips, crisps, a tin of beans, a whole jar of pickled onions or pickled anything. I'll stand in the kitchen and eat them out of the jar or tin. I have no control. Even though my stomach is full and it feels as though it's all backing up like a blocked waste-disposal system, I carry on eating. Even for normal meals I eat large, large portions.'*

After working with me, Sarah found that her whole attitude to food changed.

'Before, if someone asked, "Do you want vegetables?" I would always say, "No thank you," but since I have been seeing you, I can't get enough of my vegetables. Also, the other day there were chocolates on my boss's desk, and I realised I just didn't fancy them. I kept visualising myself at my dream size, and I just walked on by. I eat slowly now and I feel full quicker. I am listening to my body for the first time ever. It's a revelation.'

In just three months with Hypnodiet, Sarah has gone from a size 14 to a size 10.

'This is the new me. I can't believe how easy it's been.'

HypnoDIET tip
Don't settle for second best

I've heard women say, so many times, 'Well, I'd love to be a size 10', or, men have said, 'I'd love to have a 30-inch waist', and then they say, 'but realistically I'm kidding myself. I'll be happy to just be a size 12/14 [or a 34-inch waist].' Absolutely not! Women: go for the size 10! Men: go for the 30-inch waist! You can do this.

HOW TO USE YOUR VISUALISATION TOOL

Your visualisation will become part of your daily meditations, using the CD.

1   Each time you listen to the CD, take a moment to look at and study your chosen picture – your Visualisation Tool. Really focus on it – before closing your eyes.

2   When you get to the section in the CD where I ask you to imagine yourself the size you want to be, you will have that image clearly in your brain. You'll see how easy this is.

3   Listen to the CD every day and you'll be amazed at how quickly and easily you reach this 'dream' size. The fact is, it's not a dream – it's a reality. Your reality.

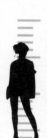

HypnoDIET tip
Keep remembering

Keep your image handy in your food diary so that when you fill in your diary each day you are constantly reminded visually of what you can achieve.

YOUR ACHIEVABLE GOAL

Creating your Visualisation Tool will give you a far more vivid goal – it will put the image into your subconscious, so that you genuinely believe that it is possible for you to become that size and shape.

It is important, from now on, to think of size and shape and not to think in terms of kilos or pounds.

> *I advise people to get rid of the bathroom scales entirely. They only lead to obsession and distress.*

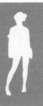

Instead of using the bathroom scales, focus on the overall size you want to be, and will be, with Hypnodiet, and enjoy the image in your mind.

No, this isn't an impossibility. I've seen it happen again and again. It will happen to you too.

WHEN WEAKNESS STRIKES, IT'S NOT ALL OVER

It's very easy to believe that you've 'blown it' if you end up overeating on one occasion; for example, at a party, or if you finish that huge bar of chocolate in the fridge or you were

Deepening your visualisation

As you look at your image, ask yourself:

- How will it feel to run my hands over my slim body?
- What it is like to imagine this slim body in the mirror and to wear my favourite style of clothes?
- How will this body feel when walking, sitting, swimming, moving around – being looked at?
- How will it feel to have a small waist, neat hips and thighs, defined shoulders and slender arms? How does it feel to enjoy a flat, toned stomach and midriff?
- Imagine you are walking across a square in a fabulous city such as Venice. You are walking across St Mark's Square with an amazing air of confidence, turning heads as you go. People having coffees on pavement cafés are watching you admiringly as you walk across the square. How does that feel? You are enjoying them watching you (probably for the first time you can remember – enjoying people looking at you).

unable to resist that enormous slice of cake. It's easy to beat yourself up when this happens, and say, 'I'll never look the way I want. I can't do it!' And then it's even easier to think, *Well, I might as well just eat the whole cake . . . I've ruined it all now.* Not any more.

Normal eating means that you *can* occasionally have a slice of cake or a piece of chocolate. People who are 'naturally slim' do have the odd treat, but if they eat too much, they also tend to compensate for this later by eating less. They don't do this because they're denying themselves food, or feeling guilty, they do it because they recognise that their body does not need or want so much.

Hypnodiet will help you to break the cycle of guilt that leads you to binge.

YOU'LL BE IN CONTROL

Hypnodiet allows you to have a treat, and then to stop. It allows you to recognise, later, that you're just not that hungry. You will, perhaps for the first time, listen to your body, and when you do this you'll gain confidence in yourself. You're in charge! You will quickly experience a real change in yourself in that you will no longer be looking for food. It will feel as though you have a new-found respect for your body – something you may never have experienced before.

By visualising yourself the way you want to be, you'll reach your goal easily, without stress or self-denial. Your mind is an incredibly powerful tool.

Using mini-visualisations

You can use your visualisation skills at any time alongside your daily meditations – while waiting for a bus, or when you're in a boring situation! Regular self-visualisation is a good way to remind yourself constantly where you are heading, and why. It only takes a moment.

1   Close your eyes. Take a deep breath in through your nose and deep into your lungs; fill your lungs with oxygen.

2   Hold for a moment, and then slowly release the breath through your mouth. Repeat this deep breathing in and out for about ten times. As you breathe in, fill your lungs with more oxygen. Regular breathing exercises help you to breathe correctly.

3   Take a moment to visualise yourself the size you want to be – to 'think yourself slim'.

4   You may instantly react to that suggestion with, 'That's impossible!' It isn't. Remember, I have helped thousands of people, just like you, to realise that 'impossibility'.

5   Enter, mindfully, into that new body: what do I look like when I look in the mirror? What clothes am I wearing? How does it feel to live in this new body?

Chapter 7

LIVE WELL

You're probably already painfully aware that being overweight isn't good for you. You probably also understand the health issues that are associated with your excess weight: the increased risk of cancer, heart disease, diabetes and joint problems, to name just a few. You probably also know, all too well, that as you age these problems are likely to become more acute. The great news is that you have done your body a huge favour by starting my programme.

This is the start of a lifestyle change that will not only make you slimmer but also healthier, happier and more energetic.

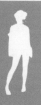

A HEALTHY WEIGHT EQUALS
IMMEDIATE BENEFITS

Research shows that losing just 5 to 10 per cent of your weight over a three-to-six-month period brings enormous health benefits, such as lowering your risk of type-2 diabetes and high blood pressure.

Hypnodiet is not just about looks, it's about how you live.

MAKING SENSE OF IT ALL

Even the best informed person can find it hard to work their way through the minefield of conflicting advice on what, when and how to eat. Open any magazine or newspaper and you're sure to find articles on 'superfoods' and dietary supplements, or reports on studies that show how this or that food now causes – or protects against – cancer, or heart disease, Alzheimer's or other major conditions. The advice and evidence seem to change from one minute to the next.

You end up confused. Then you give up even trying.

IT'S EASIER THAN YOU THINK

I always tell everyone that living well is simple. In fact, the core advice hasn't changed all that much over the years, and it's no secret how to eat well and lose inches. Most experts will probably tell you that our grandmothers knew best when they said that 'small meals and often' is a sensible approach to life. One expert famously summed it up in just eight words: 'Eat real food, not too much, mostly plants.'

Of course, when it comes down to it, you've probably found that it's not always that easy, is it? There are temptations everywhere: fast food, chocolates, ready meals, gourmet restaurants, and so on.

Well, with Hypnodiet, you are going to be able to resist those stimuli. You'll learn to eat (and still enjoy) simple, wholesome, healthy food in moderation – and you won't be denying yourself 'treats' either. You will learn to provide your body with key nutrients and to take regular exercise, as well as keeping those treats to a minimum. Best of all, you'll find this achievable and fulfilling.

> *You'll lose weight, and you'll feel amazing when you do.*

★ **Case Study:** Nicole

WHEN I FIRST SAW NICOLE, 33, who works in television, she was a good size 14 and wanted to be a size 10. But she was in despair, locked into a cycle of binge eating and dieting since her late teens.

'I hate being addicted to food and I hate being fat. I have joined a gym, but I put my trainers on and then think, Oh

why bother? I'm self-destructive, out of control. I'll carry around vitamin drinks and a packet of dried fruit and nuts but they are still in my bag when I get home. It's like I set myself up for failure.'

In our second session, Nicole talked about how she had begun to look after herself.

'I'm eating lots of fruit, and I'm eating mindfully. I was having lunch with my mum the other day and she said, "Why are you eating like that, don't you like it?" I realised that she was making comments about how slowly I was eating. I haven't been eating between meals, and the other day it was someone's birthday at work, and there were cupcakes – I have never, ever refused them before, but I just didn't feel like eating them. It was quite a revelation. I have a long way to go, but I felt firmly in control. Food is not ruling me any more.'

Nicole reached her target weight in four months, and has stayed that way for two years now. Her story still makes me cry. Not just for Nicole, but for the many hundreds of people with similar experiences whom I have listened to over the years.

THE SIMPLE RULES

My advice on living well is to follow some simple rules. I've outlined these opposite. Your daily meditations will help you to stick to them.

RULE 1: GET MOVING

A cornerstone of my method is exercise. Hypnodiet helps you to embrace exercise rather than seeing it as a chore. Exercise will become an essential part of your daily life, not an optional extra. As well as helping with weight control, it gives you energy and improves your mood. With regular exercise, your body shape and composition will change: your muscles will become more toned and dense and will therefore burn calories quicker.

MOVE YOUR BODY, FEED YOUR MIND

The improvements in your mood can be life-changing in themselves. When you exercise, your body releases endorphins – these are the so-called 'feel-good hormones'. Endorphins give you a natural high, so exercise, quite literally, can make you feel happy. And when you feel happy you are less likely to turn to food for comfort or solace.

WALKING TO WELL-BEING

I always tell my clients that one of the best all-round forms of exercise is walking. You don't need any equipment, and it's free. Anyone can do it, and it can be really enjoyable. Walking is the most natural and fundamental of all conscious movements, but we underestimate its invaluable contribution to our health and well-being.

Aim to walk for 30 minutes, at least five days a week. This

may sound intimidating if you're new to exercise, but it doesn't have to be. The good news is that you don't have to do your walking in one block of time. In fact, recent studies show that brisk walking in 5 to 10-minute bursts throughout your day is just as effective as working out for 30 minutes in the gym.

If you can build walking into your daily life, it's likely to be more sustainable – walking to work, for example, instead of driving, or getting off the bus a few stops before your destination, then walking the extra 10 minutes at a good pace. This takes planning and thought, but you will see the benefits. Your daily meditations, on the accompanying CD, will help you to instinctively prioritise this, even to crave it.

TREADING PURPOSEFULLY

If you prefer to work out using equipment, I always advocate power walking on a treadmill. I have a treadmill at home and have been walking this way for years – virtually every gym has them too. My treadmill is vital to my well-being. I love my daily sessions. As I walk, I listen to my music; I always choose music with an upbeat tempo – this helps me to power walk. I lose myself in my imagination and it makes me feel amazing. It truly is 'me time' and it fits perfectly into my busy schedule. I exercise for around 20 to 30 minutes each day – invariably after I have finished work. However, I do believe that first thing in the morning is the best time to exercise, if possible. I do this at weekends and holidays, but I never have the time during the working week.

You need to aim for a fast pace – the kind of speed you'd walk if you were late for an appointment. You may be slightly out of breath, warm, but able to carry on a basic conversation.

> *When it comes to exercise, do whatever fits into your busy life.*

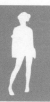

Hypno DIET tip
Walking the pounds away

Experts advise finding your 'optimum walking pace'. To do this, speed up your walking until you find the point at which you have to break into a jog. Your 'optimum walking pace' is about 5–10 per cent slower than this. At this pace, you will get the maximum cardiovascular benefit from walking. The pace is fast, but not punishing. Take long strides.

Walking this way firms and lifts the buttocks, and tones the thighs and the backs of the legs. Swinging your arms at the same pace as you walk can help to firm up your middle back and the upper arms, either getting rid of those 'bingo wings' or making sure that you don't get them in the first place!

CHOOSE CAREFULLY

Many people, when they try to lose weight and get fit, launch into strenuous routines. They want rapid results – to be fitter, stronger, toned and powerful – so they sign up to boot camps, join gyms and start aerobics classes. Like diets, this may work for a while, but it is rarely sustainable.

Most people don't have access to personal trainers or have five hours a day to spend doing high-impact exercise routines. But we can all walk. You may also wish to combine walking with other forms of exercise – whether strenuous or gentle: an exercise ball, yoga classes, team sports or swimming, for example. All of these activities will enhance your well-being. But you don't have to do anything elaborate. Walking is a miracle exercise in its own right. And it's one you can start today and continue for the rest of your life, whatever shape you're in.

HypnoDIET tip

What you're aiming for

Government health advisers say that we should all aim to walk about 10,000 steps per day, but most of us don't get anywhere near this. It takes a bit of planning, but it's perfectly achievable if you build short spurts of walking into your day. I always advise, along with many other experts, getting a pedometer so that you can track your steps. Walking an extra 5,000 steps a day can burn off 1,240 calories over a week. Walking is an excellent fitness tool.

Five healthy exercising habits

1 Always walk briskly whenever you can, rather than taking the car or bus. Even short bursts of activity are immensely effective.

2 Energetic housework or gardening will count as part of your daily activity.

3 Change your daily habits: stand up while talking on the telephone, get up during the advert breaks when watching TV and move around, run up the stairs rather than walking. Small changes can have big results.

4 Take lunch breaks! At work take a ten-minute walk around the block at lunchtime. Use the stairs, not the lift.

5 Get an 'exercise buddy' (a friend who you can walk, jog or play sport with). If you have a dog, be eager to take him or her for a brisk daily walk.

HOW WILL YOU GET MOTIVATED?

You may be feeling intimidated by all this talk of exercise – well don't be! Through the meditations I will teach you to embrace walking – and any form of exercise you choose. Rather than seeing exercise as a chore, you will soon come to

Exercise will soon become something you love to do.

view activity as an essential part of your life – something you simply can't live without!

RULE 2: EAT WELL

It's important to understand some basics about how to eat well: nothing faddy, just sensible, sustainable changes that will help you to feel and look amazing. Eating well isn't complicated and it isn't hard to achieve. Here is my basic guide. For a balanced diet, try to:

- Eat plenty of fruit, vegetables and wholegrain carbohydrates (for example, wholemeal bread, brown rice and wholewheat pasta).
- Have smaller amounts of milk and dairy products (go for lower fat versions where possible) and eat smaller amounts of lean meat. (See Getting the Portions Right on page 49.)
- Limit sugary food and fats – these are often your treats, which you don't want to let go of yet!
- Limit bad fats; that is, saturated fats and avoid trans-fats. (For more information, see page 113.)

FRUIT AND VEGETABLES

You probably already know that you should be eating five portions of fruit and vegetables every day at the very least (in some countries the advice is to eat ten portions of fruit and vegetables a day!). There is a huge amount of scientific research showing that people whose diets are rich in fruit and vegetables have a much lower risk of cancers and other serious illnesses. Fruit and vegetables also contain dietary fibre, which can help weight control, as it gives a fuller feeling. And they are rich in antioxidants, which help cell renewal – keeping you looking and feeling younger.

Fruit and vegetables are powerhouses of nutrients that will help you feel fit and well.

My top three fruit and vegetable tips

1 **Eat foods rich in vitamin E every day**. This antioxidant vitamin has been proven to lower the risk of heart disease and some cancers. It is also often used in skin creams and lotions, because it slows down the cell ageing process, and topically for injuries such as burns, because it accelerates the healing process and reduces scarring. **Good sources** are vegetable oils such as olive oil (go for cold-pressed extra virgin where you can), sunflower oil, wheatgerm oil and corn oil; nuts (such as almonds, hazelnuts and peanuts), sunflower seeds, avocados, tomatoes, kiwi fruit, wholegrains, leafy green vegetables, blackberries and mangoes.

2   **Eat plenty of berries**. Berries are antioxidant rich and high in vitamin C. Try sprinkling them on porridge at breakfast time, taking them to work as snacks or eating them with low-fat natural yoghurt as a dessert. They are also delicious (especially blueberries), sprinkled over a stir-fry.

Choose from cherries, blueberries, blackberries, strawberries or raspberries.

3   **Eat your greens**. Leafy greens such as spinach or kale are rich in folic acid and vitamin B$_6$, which helps to produce serotonin – a brain chemical that boosts your mood and alertness, and plays a role in controlling your sleep cycles. Reliable research shows that broccoli and other 'cruciferous' vegetables (vegetables whose leaves form a cross) have fantastic anti-cancer properties.

Make sure you eat broccoli, spinach, cauliflower, Brussels sprouts and cabbage.

HypnoDIET tip

Veggie snacks

Keep bags of chopped raw vegetables in the fridge and take them in your bag as snacks for the day. They are surprisingly yummy when eaten raw.

NOT ALL FATS ARE EQUAL

You may have come to believe that all dietary fats are forbidden if you want to get thinner. You probably think that fat makes you FAT. Dietary fat is certainly calorie dense, but certain kinds – such as olive oil or the fats found in nuts and seeds – have huge health benefits. Indeed, they can actually help you to lose weight.

It's important to understand the difference between 'good fats', which should be a daily part of your diet, and 'bad fats', which can be harmful to the body. Bad fats should be avoided (or at least kept to a minimum – I am aware that you may find it difficult never to eat cheese or a cake again, for example).

GOOD FATS The body needs a certain amount of essential fatty acids. These are extremely good for the heart and play a crucial role in brain function and the development of healthy brain cells. Omega-3 oils are one major type of essential fatty acid, and extensive research has shown that they are a vital part of a healthy diet. They are found in oily fish, such as salmon, sardines and mackerel.

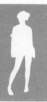

Aim to eat fish at least twice a week to boost your body's intake of omega-3 oils.

Omega-3 oils are also found in walnuts, omega-3-enriched eggs, rapeseed and soya oils. Try using rapeseed oil in salad dressings, sprinkle walnuts on your cereal or salads and eat plenty of green, leafy vegetables. (Store rapeseed oil in the fridge.)

A healthy diet should also include omega-6 fatty acids, but most diets already provide more than enough of these. They are found in vegetable oils such as sunflower, corn and soya oil and spreads made from them. If you are eating low-fat spreads, do check they do not contain trans-fats (see below for more about trans-fats).

BAD FATS Saturates are types of fat found in animal products (butter, cheese and meats), cakes, biscuits and pastries. This kind of fat raises your risk of heart disease, and is never going to help your waistline! I always advise people to cut out or cut down on saturates wherever possible. Switch from butter to low-fat spread, cut off visible fat from meat and poultry, and choose lower fat meat and dairy products where you can.

Trans-fats are another type of bad fat, which you should avoid. They are known to increase your risk of heart disease and also certain cancers. They are found mostly in crackers, crisps and mass-produced biscuits and cakes, although they are sometimes also found in low-fat spreads too, so keep an eye on labels. Trans-fats are produced artificially in a high-temperature process called hydrogenation, which turns liquid fat into solid fat, giving the product a longer shelf life and making it spreadable. It is cheap to manufacture. There is an overwhelming scientific case and urgency for trans-fats to be banned from foods, and most retailers are doing this, but until they are banned completely I always advise people to check labels and avoid foods containing them.

Note

CHOOSE LOW-FAT DAIRY PRODUCTS: SEMI-SKIMMED OR SKIMMED MILK, REDUCED-FAT CHEESE, LOW-FAT YOGHURT OR FROMAGE FRAIS. CHANGING TO SEMI-SKIMMED MILK CAN SAVE YOU AROUND 60 CALORIES PER DAY – OR 420 CALORIES OVER A WEEK, IF YOU USUALLY CONSUME ABOUT 300ML (10FL OZ/½ PINT) OF MILK PER DAY.

WHOLEGRAIN CARBOHYDRATES

Brown rice, wholemeal bread and wholewheat pastas are all types of wholegrain carbohydrates, which release energy more slowly than refined carbohydrates, such as bread made with white flour, white rice or white pasta. This simply means that they keep you feeling fuller for longer. Wholegrain foods help you to avoid that blood-sugar rush, followed by the sugar crash, which then, usually, has you

craving for something sweet or energy boosting, like a chocolate bar or a chunk of cheese.

Brown rice is an excellent wholegrain food to use as a
base for some of your meals. It contains vitamins, proteins
and minerals, and tastes delicious.

I never advise cutting out carbohydrates completely, but I
do believe it's a good idea to switch to wholegrains wherever
you can, and to eat them in moderation.

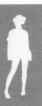

> *Eat wholegrain carbs. They
> provide sustained energy rather
> than a quick boost followed
> by a sugar crash.*

Getting the idea

I don't believe in diets, but I do believe in healthy eating and
the occasional treat. Eat the four basics: fruit, vegetables, fish
and chicken (or vegetarian alternatives: beans, lentils, nuts
and tofu, for example). If you prefer to have some idea
about meals, here are some sample menus:

Day 1

Breakfast 2 eggs, scrambled or as an omelette; small
seasonal fresh fruit salad with fresh lime squeezed
over and drizzled with honey

Lunch   Thick lentil soup; one small slice of rye bread; small prawn, grapefruit and avocado salad

Dinner   Grilled chicken breast drizzled with olive oil; small baked sweet potato; lightly steamed spinach and walnuts; chocolate mousse

Day 2

Breakfast Porridge sprinkled with blueberries, raspberries or strawberries

Lunch   Avocado and chicken salad; multigrain bread with flaxseeds; tropical fruit: sliced mango, pineapple or papaya

Dinner   Poached salmon; lightly steamed asparagus with freshly squeezed lemon juice

Snacks

Select one snack for mid-morning and one for mid-afternoon:

    Nuts: almonds, walnuts

    Piece of fruit

    Small chunk of cheese

    Small handful of black grapes

    Few squares of chocolate

A word about dietary supplements

It's common for people on a 'health kick' to visit the health-food shop and buy lots of dietary supplements in the hope that this will give them all the nutrients they need. This is not just a huge expense – it also gives you a false sense of security.

Despite a massive food-supplements industry, there is conflicting scientific evidence that vitamin pills actually work. The combination of different nutrients in the body, rather than the individual vitamins themselves, is what's crucial to our health. A daily multivitamin won't do any harm as a basic insurance policy, but it is mistaken to rely on supplements alone. Skipping meals or eating badly won't be OK just because you've had a handful of vitamins during the day. In short, you will get the most benefit by eating a variety of healthy foods, including the widest range of fresh fruit and vegetables, pulses (peas, beans and lentils), nuts, seeds, eggs and oily fish, with lean meat occasionally.

RULE 3: DRINK WELL

Drink more water! Most people are woefully dehydrated. You should aim to drink at least eight glasses of water every day. Water helps your digestion – ensuring regular bowel movements – clears your skin and boosts your general well-being. (Dehydration is energy sapping and can bring your mood down and cause headaches.)

I advise people to start every day with hot water and lemon in order to kick-start the digestion. After this, drink water – as much as possible – throughout the day. It's surprising how easy it is to confuse thirst with hunger.

Note

BE AWARE THAT DRINKING WATER THROUGHOUT THE DAY AT REGULAR INTERVALS IS GOOD, BUT DRINKING SAY 3–4 LITRES (5¼–7 PINTS) OR MORE IN ONE GO IS DANGEROUS. NOT ONLY DOES IT FLUSH OUT YOUR NATURAL MINERALS AND SALTS AS WELL AS ANY MEDICATION YOU MAY BE TAKING BUT IT CAN ALSO KILL YOU!

OTHER DRINKS

Apart from water, choose herbal teas such as green tea: this is a natural weight-loss aid that stimulates the fat-burning process. It also has antioxidant properties that support the immune system.

Try to wean yourself off cordials, as they contain a surprising number of calories. It's also worth knowing that fruit juices can give you the blood-sugar 'spikes' you are trying to steer clear of.

Avoid 'diet fizzy drinks', as they are not diet aids at all and they contain artificial sweeteners. Naturally sweetened foods and drinks are far better than artificially sweetened ones. It's also amazing how many 'empty' calories can come from a fizzy drink or cordial habit.

If you enjoy fruit juices, have these just once a day, diluted with water, as they are a concentrated form of sugar, which can create a blood-sugar rush followed by a dip. Blood-sugar highs and lows are not good for weight loss.

> *Drink water for clear skin and good health. Avoid fizzy drinks offering little nutritious value.*

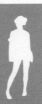

ALCOHOL

If you are one of many who enjoy a glass of wine or beer at the end of the day, and for most days, try to keep it to a minimum and drink slowly. It's a good idea to pour yourself a small glass rather than a large one (have you noticed how wine glasses in restaurants and bars are huge these days?). Not only can alcohol contribute to weight gain but it can also store up health problems (breast and oesophageal cancers, for example, are directly linked to alcohol consumption). So, try to keep well within the government limits – that's 14 units a week for women, 21 units for men. It may surprise you to know that one large glass of wine – the size many people pour themselves these days – can contain as many as 4 units of alcohol. A pint of standard beer, meanwhile, has 2 units of alcohol and 182 calories – fine if it's the odd one, but not great if you are trying to control your waistline!

HypnoDIET tip
For chocolate lovers

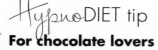

Research shows that there are more antioxidants in pure cocoa powder than red wine and green tea. This doesn't mean you should gorge on chocolate; if you do, you'll find it very hard to lose weight, but the odd square of high-cocoa-content, dark chocolate certainly won't do you any harm, and may even do some good!

Five healthy eating habits

1 Eat breakfast (see Chapter 3, page 47).
2 Eat three meals every day – plan these in advance when possible (see page 55).
3 Eat at the table, without distractions such as TV or reading. Enjoy your food.
4 Serve your food on smaller plates.
5 Eat slowly and chew your food well: about 12–14 times.

HEALTHY SNACKING

Snacks are invaluable for balancing blood-sugar levels and staving off hunger, but foods such as crisps, biscuits, chocolate and sweets – the kind of thing you'll find in rail stations and corner shops when you're on the hop – are all high in 'bad' fats, sugar or salt. Eaten occasionally in small amounts won't do you any harm, but mostly you want to choose snacks that give you energy, vitamins and minerals without too much fat, sugar or salt. This way your snacks will enhance rather than diminish your health.

Healthy snacks help you get through the day and feel great.

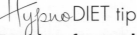

HypnoDIET tip
Top ideas for good snacking

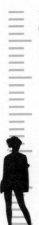

- Keep fruit handy where it's easy to grab if you're peckish.
- Take a bag of chopped fruit or raw vegetables, such as carrot sticks, to work, so that you don't find yourself at the vending machine when you're hungry.
- Try to include some protein in your snacks – a handful of nuts (go for plain, not roasted or salted), a small piece of cheese or a slice of lean meat. This will help to keep you feeling satisfied for longer.

SNACK IDEAS

If you plan ahead for snacks you'll be less likely to grab something unhealthy when you're desperate:

1   Small bowl of wholegrain cereal with semi-skimmed milk.
2   Slice of wholegrain toast with low-fat cheese spread and a tomato.
3   A banana and a few walnuts.
4   Carrot and celery sticks with cottage cheese or low-fat hummus.
5   Dried apricots or other dried fruit, with a couple of Brazil nuts.
6   Low-fat yoghurt. (Many of us don't get enough calcium; low-fat natural yoghurt is a good way of boosting your intake.)
7   Two oatcakes with peanut butter.

Banana power

Recent research has proved the health benefits of eating bananas regularly. They are high in potassium and low in salt, and also contain magnesium, vitamins B_6 and B_{12}, iron and fibre. Eating bananas regularly can cut the risk of fatal strokes by as much as 40 per cent, and they can also help you relax, as well as improving your mood and generally making you feel happier, This is because they contain tryptophan: a protein that the body converts into serotonin, the feel-good chemical. The potassium in the fruit can also boost your brainpower, assist learning and make you feel more alert. So bananas are a useful fruit to eat as part of your healthy diet.

TOP WAYS TO LIVE WELL

Here is a summary of my top tips for feeling great and looking good. Keep them to hand as you start to implement the Hypnodiet.

1   **Make exercise a part of your life** – whether it's walking on a treadmill, around your office block at lunchtime or walking your dog in the park, taking a yoga class, working out in the gym or fitting in a daily swim. Whatever it is, the key is to do it, and do it daily. (Walking is easy and it brings maximum health benefits – and just about everyone can manage it.)

2   **Slow down and eat mindfully** (see Chapter 3 for a full explanation of mindful eating).

3   **Plan your menus.** This will help you to include fruit and vegetables – ideally lots – in every meal. Switch to

wholegrains, and have healthy snacks at the ready.
Turn back to pages 122–3 for further healthy snacks.

4   **Eat regular meals.** Try to sit down to eat at roughly
the same times each day, and don't skip meals. Studies
show that those who eat a good, healthy breakfast
every day control their weight better than those who
skip it.

5   **Eat good fats.** Cut down on saturates (for example,
switch to low-fat dairy products) but include
moderate amounts of heart-healthy fats such as
omega-3 and omega-6 (although avoid hydrogenated
margarines with trans-fats).

6   **Drink more water.** Take a bottle of water with you
wherever you go: keep one on your desk, take one
when you go shopping, and refill your glass
throughout the day. You're aiming for at least eight
glasses a day, but ideally more.

7   **Control your alcohol consumption.** If you like a glass
of wine, that's fine, but keep a strict eye on your
measures and drink slowly and mindfully, and you
will extend the pleasure. Each burst of flavour is the
same, whether you take a sip or a gulp of wine. So
you will have more exciting bursts of flavour by
drinking slowly.

8   **Be more active.** Look for ways to move about
whenever you can. Take the stairs rather than the lift,

walk rather than drive to the corner shop, get off the bus before your destination and walk. Even just standing up on the tube, train, bus, and so on, burns an extra 70 calories an hour. When you are watching TV try to get up during the ad breaks – do a few chores, put the dishes in the dishwasher, or put the rubbish out. Any activity is good!

Hypno DIET tip

Liven up your food the healthy way

Use freshly squeezed lime or lemon juice on fruit, fish and vegetables. It's delicious and much better for you than heavy sauces containing butter or cream. Just try it.

EATING OUT

Having a meal out is part of modern life. Hypnodiet will help you to make good, healthy choices when in a restaurant, just as you would at home or in the supermarket. You will also be more mindful regarding portion sizes and even enjoy eating out.

> *With Hypnodiet, you will no longer feel anxious about eating out.*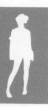

WATCH THOSE RESTAURANT PORTIONS

Restaurant portions are invariably too generous, particularly in this supersize era. So, try to size up your food before you eat, and use this simple method: a sensible portion of meat is the size of a small chicken breast; a sensible cheese portion is two slithers just to taste; a portion of dried pasta or rice is the size of a small tea cup. If your portions are supersized, simply cut them down before you begin eating and put the excess to one side of the plate.

HOW IT'S COOKED ACTUALLY MATTERS

When ordering, it's a good idea to think about the way the food is cooked. Where possible, choose foods that are steamed, poached, roasted, grilled or baked rather than fried, cooked au gratin (sprinkled with breadcrumbs and/or cheese), breaded or creamed.

DRESSING DOWN

A salad can make a great starter or a main, but don't assume that because it's green it's healthy. Salads – not to mention vegetable side dishes – can come with rich dressings or sauces that turn a healthy meal into a fat-soaked binge. I tend to ask for simple French-style dressings on the side so that I can put a small amount on the salad myself. Ask for your vegetables to come steamed, without butter, too. Simple choices like these can turn a blowout into a delicious, but healthy, dining experience.

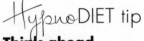 **DIET tip**

Think ahead

If you know that you are going to be eating out that evening, just eat normally throughout the day and don't be tempted to think you have to starve yourself so that you can 'pig out' at dinner. Hypnodiet doesn't work like that. Dinner is just another meal – it may be in a fabulous restaurant, but it's just another meal. If you starve yourself in the day and you go to the restaurant ravenous, you'll just be tempted to overeat and regret it later.

LET HYPNODIET TAKE THE STRAIN

So, this is the formula you need to make changes, but the real key is motivation: making healthy changes that will last for the rest of your life. Your daily Hypnodiet meditations will give you the tools to do this. None of it will be painful or involve huge amounts of willpower.

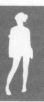

You will find the motivation to make healthy changes – permanently.

KEEPING IT SIMPLE

Making lifestyle changes doesn't have to be complicated. Soon you'll find it comes as second nature to choose fruit instead of biscuits, to walk to work, to sprinkle nuts on your salad, to have a small glass of wine, then stop.

You'll wonder how you ever lived any other way.

Chapter 8

HOW TO GET STARTED

'␣ve explained all the elements that make up a healthy lifestyle, which you can kick-start by following the Hypnodiet meditations. Now, here's your handy step-by-step guide to putting it all together so that you get fit and healthy and be happy. Many of the points have been touched upon earlier but repetition is the key to ensuring success.

GET READY

There are just a few things you need to prepare in advance, then you're ready to go. It's especially important to take the time to create your Visualisation Tool so that it's just the way you want it to be, as it will give you the inspiration for continuing success.

1   Put away your bathroom scales (page 96).
2   Create your Visualisation Tool (page 92).

3   Record the meditation CD onto your iPod or MP3 player, if you like, so that you can continue to meditate each day, even if you are away.

4   Have an exercise book or journal ready that you can use as a food diary (page 52).

PREPARE FOR THE MEDITATION

Now you have everything to hand, decide which time of the day is best for your meditation and make it a habit.

1   Set aside about 20 minutes *each* day until you reach your ideal size, and then listen to the CD just once or twice a week to maintain your new figure. Find a regular time that suits you.

2   Find a quiet spot away from distractions, but do not be over-concerned about background noise (page 68).

3   Have your Visualisation Tool handy.

4   Put the CD on the CD player and get ready to start.

5   Focus on the your Visualisation Tool before you close your eyes.

Feel the benefit from even the first meditation.

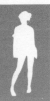

6 Close your eyes.

7 Now listen to the meditation, following my instructions.

BUILDING ON YOUR MEDITATIONS

Now you're getting into the swing of the meditations, think about how you can get more out of them.

1 After you have used the CD a few times, deepen your visualisation, if you like, by following my tip on page 97.

2 Use my mini-visualisation on page 99 whenever you are just sitting or standing around waiting.

As the days go by, you'll be feeling a great sense of achievement.

ENJOY YOUR MEALS

When the food you are eating is good, wholesome and full of natural flavours, your whole body will be thanking you. You'll be discovering how food should really taste and you'll enjoy feeling satisfied without feeling guilty.

1   Eat a healthy breakfast every day (page 47).

2   Plan your remaining two meals for the day, plus two healthy snacks. Include the healthy choices and avoid the danger foods (those high in saturated fat and/or sugar or white carbs) (page 110).

3   Eat at the table.

4   Give your food your full attention.

5   Enjoy your food, and eat to satisfy your hunger.

6   Eat 'mindfully' (Chapter 7):

  • Appreciate what you are eating.
  • Really taste your food.
  • Chew your food.
  • Think about how you feel as you eat it.

7   Stop eating when you've reached that 'had enough to eat' feeling.

8   Keep your food diary: write down *everything* you eat and drink each day and the physical activity you take – *at the time* (page 52). Write down your

In the past, emotions probably triggered off comfort eating – but not any more.

emotions and you will be able to see how patterns have developed between food and your feelings.

Note

IF YOU EAT OUT, CHOOSE SENSIBLY, AND DON'T EAT ALL THE FOOD ON YOUR PLATE IF THE PORTIONS ARE LARGE. DON'T STARVE YOURSELF DURING THE DAY IN PREPARATION FOR A BLOWOUT AT THE RESTAURANT.

KEEP HYDRATED

Drinking plenty of water or herbal teas will keep your body feeling good. If you weren't drinking enough before, you have probably lived with the constant uncomfortable effects of dehydration. Now, you'll want to benefit from everything that your body needs.

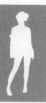

Enjoy the clear and fresh feeling from drinking plenty of water.

1   Drink plenty of water – about eight glasses each day.
2   Avoid all fizzy drinks, even diet drinks, and drink diluted fruit juices only occasionally.
3   Make alcohol an occasional treat, but only have one small glass.

KEEP EXERCISING

Take your daily exercise, and aim for 30 minutes' vigorous exercise, such as brisk walking, at least five days a week (Chapter 7).

Don't lose your resolve

Everyone has times when they feel their resolve slipping, or when they doubt whether Hypnodiet can possibly work for them. When this happens, try these motivation tips:

Tip 1: remember your reasons for losing weight
Remind yourself why you want to lose weight: is it for your health? Or for your appearance, your relationship, your self-esteem, your work – or all of these?

Tip 2: remember your achievements
Remind yourself what you've achieved so far: even the smallest steps – buying this book, for example – are important!

Tip 3: it's OK to lapse occasionally

Remember that small lapses are not the end of the world: it's OK to have a day when you feel more hungry, or a meal when you eat too much. It happens to us all. It is normal. It does not mean Hypnodiet isn't working for you. You can do this. Simply carry on with the meditations, and have faith. Hypnodiet does work and it will work for you.

BE INSPIRED

I hope that this chapter has shown you how simple it is to get started. But before you begin, read through the following chapter to discover how your life will change and how others have been inspired by a new life after using Hypnodiet.

Chapter 9

LIFE STARTS HERE

You should now have a clear idea of how hypnosis works on your mind and what Hypnodiet can do for you. Hypnodiet can bring dramatic changes to your body – benefiting the way you eat and look after yourself, and its principles can become a natural part of your everyday life.

Once you have started Hypnodiet and enjoyed all the freedom it brings, you will find that it is easy to live healthily – because that is what you will want to do. It won't be a hassle; there won't be guilt involved or depression because you feel you have failed. You will thrive on the success you are achieving day by day. It will be part of your life. Simply by making your meditations a regular habit and following my basic recommendations, dieting will be a thing of the past. Healthy eating and living will be your present and future.

Now, I hope, you will have a simple and clear understanding of what you are aiming for when it comes to planning a healthy diet and making exercise an enjoyable and essential part of your daily life, rather than an optional extra. Beginning a healthy lifestyle is straightforward and inspiring when you use the guidance of the meditations on the CD.

FIND CONFIDENCE – NOW!

You will start to feel the changes in your behaviour and attitude as soon as you've had your first Hypnodiet meditation. Hypnodiet promotes a mindful awareness to change your attitude towards food – and it works instantly.

As you continue with Hypnodiet, you will see many more changes over the coming weeks and months. You'll be able to fit into clothes you've only dreamed of wearing in the past. But that's not all; you'll also find that your posture – the way you move and hold yourself – will change too. I have noticed that no matter how tall a person is, when they feel overweight they tend to slouch. They want to hide. But when you look good and feel lean, you want to show your body to the world.

You'll develop what I call that amazingly confident 'to be seen' look. You know when people have it – they stand and

You'll find that you actually enjoy turning heads.

walk with shoulders back, head up. People's eyes are drawn to them regardless of their age or how conventionally good-looking they may or may not be. This will happen to you too.

EMBRACE THAT NEW FEELING OF SELF-ASSURANCE

When people watch you go by, you'll no longer feel intimidated. You'll no longer dread walking past a crowded café or through a busy restaurant. Quite the contrary: you will enjoy it. In short, you'll feel empowered by your new shape and your new-found confidence.

It's not just about losing the inches; with Hypnodiet, you'll have more energy, your skin will glow, and your hair will shine, you'll look and feel younger. People might even ask if you've been on holiday. I've seen and heard all of this, time and time again.

Easy tips for the new you

- It's OK to eat the occasional ice cream – go for the sugar-free variety, or just have one scoop and enjoy.
- Keep a jug of water with lemon wedges in the fridge and aim to drink it all during the day.
- Whichever way you snap it, biscuits are high in fat, carbs, sugar and calories, so there are other snacks that are much better for you. An occasional plain biscuit will not harm you, although it's best to break the biscuit habit.

- When you decide to eat just one biscuit, or a cube or two of good-quality chocolate, etc, you will savour the moment.
- It's no secret how to lose inches, it's just about being more mindful.
- If you decide to have steak and chips, eat slowly, enjoy your food and don't feel bad – but just eat healthy, clean foods for the next few days to balance it out.
- Add a handful of blueberries to salads, stir-fries, porridge and other dishes. All berries are good for you. You can add other fruits, such as mango, to sweet and savoury dishes.
- Move at every opportunity – clench your buttocks while standing, sitting, watching TV, waiting to get on a plane, and so on. Do leg lifts while watching TV.
- Love your body, whether it's slim or not quite perfect for you. Enjoy it. Hypnodiet will help you to have a body you will feel proud of.
- Stop obsessing about your body size, and whether you look fat in certain clothes. Look forward to the new you.
- Eat lots of greens – they are bursting with health benefits. When eaten lightly steamed or stir-fried, leafy greens retain their freshness and taste great with a little seasoning, a small knob of butter and perhaps a little chopped mint or mint sauce.
- Freeze fruit and then liquidise it to make a tasty sorbet.
- Eat your five-a-day now! Don't wait to be diagnosed with a medical condition to make you do it.

SUCCESS IS JUST AROUND THE CORNER

You no longer need to feel trapped in a body that makes you feel so unhappy and even angry, as Mary has discovered.

★ **Case study:** Mary.

MARY IS A GP IN HER LATE TWENTIES. When she first came to see me she was a size 16 and wanted to be a size 10. Until she was 18 years old, she'd been a size 8, but then she was diagnosed with polycystic ovaries and had gained weight ever since. Mary had tried every fad diet going and had virtually given up until her friend came to see me and dropped three dress sizes. Mary was bored with people saying that she was pretty apart from her weight, and tired of her mother saying, 'You'll be a stunner when you lose weight.' She hadn't had a relationship since her early twenties, and she couldn't even bring herself to go shopping any more. Her mother complained that she'd become loud and aggressive.

'It's true. I have become aggressive. I feel angry. I obsess about eating and I feel like a failure.'

After two sessions with me, and over a five-month period, Mary reached her target size. She's stayed slim for two years now and says her whole life has been transformed.

'I'm not angry any more. I feel liberated.'

YOUR LIFE CAN CHANGE

I've worked with countless people who have turned their lives around as they lose their preoccupation with food. Think of all the time and mental energy you waste thinking about what you should and shouldn't eat. From now on, all that energy can be used for other, far more important, things. Clients of mine have changed careers, taken up activities they'd always wanted to try, ended or begun relationships or thrown themselves into new projects – all kick-started by Hypnodiet.

> *Hypnodiet doesn't just change the way the world sees you – it changes the way you see the world.*

★ **Case study:** Nicole

NICOLE, 36, IS AN IT MANAGER. She told me:

'I find the hypnosis CD you gave me to play between sessions of hypnosis makes me so calm. I also completed my food diary every day and really enjoyed doing it. I have used food diaries before, but not like this, where I related food to my emotions. I didn't realise how stressful my job is until I started to write it down each day in my diary.

'I haven't had any takeaways and have not snacked unhealthily once. I have been much more conscious of how

thirsty I have been and have drunk lots of water. I've also
noticed that my fridge is full of what I call "clean food" . . .
and my husband has also commented on this. He always
eats healthily, as he trains for marathons, so he is delighted
with my new healthy regime. He has seen me go through so
many diets, but he said that this time I am different and
very driven. It's as though I have my own agenda and
nothing will get in my way.

'I'm eating much slower and feeling full. One day we
went to a barbecue. In the past I would have eaten as much
as I could, then felt bad and given up on the diet. I would
have got cross with myself for not looking after my body
and with drinking too much alcohol. This time I was
absolutely fine and thought, Hey ho, tomorrow's a new
day. Although I did briefly feel I had let myself down, the
feeling soon passed!

'We went to my parents' for Sunday lunch and my
brother and sister were there with their families. It is a
rare occurrence for all of us to be together other than for
special occasions. Usually, I dread it as far as eating is
concerned, as I tend to adhere to my old childhood routine
of overeating and shovelling my food down in the race to
get second helpings, but, amazingly, I didn't this time. I
ate what everyone else was eating, but I had smaller
portions. My husband is the only one I have told about
this programme, so he is in my support group, and we

smiled to each other when he realised my delight at eating sensibly. I am having a ball in so many ways since I started this programme.'

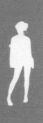

'I couldn't believe that it was so easy . . . I look at my friends, still worried all the time about their weight, and I feel sorry for them.'

★ **Case Study:** Samantha

WHEN SAMANTHA, 30, an actress, came to see me she was a size 14 but wanted to be a size 8.

'I've tried so many diets – I have a wardrobe of clothes in so many different sizes.'

She told me that she'd heard about me from a friend who had 'amazingly lost loads of weight', kept it off and was so happy.

'I want to be realistic. I want to eat the occasional burger, ice cream and chocolate and get drunk on a Saturday night – but I don't want to get upset about it. I don't want to be a gym fanatic either.'

Samantha's problems go right back to childhood. At school and college there was huge peer pressure to be slim. She gained a little weight at college, and her parents attacked her for being overweight:

'They seemed to watch every mouthful I ate and would either comment, "Should you be eating that?" or give me "the look", then I would actually eat more.

'Part of me wanted to be slim, and yet there was a little voice inside my head sabotaging all of this. It seemed to be saying, "You can do it next week or next month or for your next holiday, so just eat what you want now and it will make you happy, and you can sort it out later."

'I knew that when I was slim I felt happier, and I got more work as an actress. I knew that looks and body shape are very important in my industry. I also got more attention from guys – I think this is because I feel better about myself when I am slim, so I am more confident.'

Like many people, Samantha was well informed about what she should and shouldn't be eating.

'I feel I know so much about nutrition – I'm a magazine junkie and I'm always tearing out the latest diet or nutrition tips. But I'm so tired of the obsession.'

Hypnodiet liberated her from all that. She began to see that she could eat moderate amounts of food, with the odd treat, integrate exercise into her day by walking everywhere, and swimming at her local pool – and she felt amazing. When she reached her size 8, just eight months later, she told me:

'I couldn't believe that it was so easy. I never felt deprived, and best of all I lost that feeling of anxiety and guilt – I *found that I actually craved healthy food. I didn't even want to get drunk at the weekends. It was like this huge weight was lifted. I know I'll eat this way for life. I look at my friends, still worried all the time about their weight, and I feel sorry for them.'*

TIME TO MAKE IT HAPPEN

So now it's over to you. Use my CD for your daily meditations and start writing in your food diary today. Re-read this book, or selected chapters, whenever you want inspiration, ideas or clarification. You are now one of thousands of people who have turned their lives around with Hypnodiet.

It starts right here, right now. Enjoy it!

Index